Emergency Care of Minor Trauma in Children

D1380702

Emergency Care of Minor Trauma in Children
Third Edition

Ffion Davies
Consultant in Emergency Medicine
University Hospitals of Leicester
Leicester, United Kingdom

Colin E. Bruce
Consultant Orthopaedic and Trauma Surgeon
Alder Hey Children's Hospital
Liverpool, United Kingdom

Kate Taylor-Robinson
Consultant Paediatric Radiologist
Alder Hey Children's Hospital
Liverpool, United Kingdom

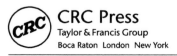

CRC Press
Taylor & Francis Group
Boca Raton London New York

CRC Press is an imprint of the
Taylor & Francis Group, an **informa** business

CRC Press
Taylor & Francis Group
6000 Broken Sound Parkway NW, Suite 300
Boca Raton, FL 33487-2742

International Standard Book Number-13: 978-1-4987-8771-0 (Paperback); 978-1-138-04829-4 (Hardback)

Library of Congress Cataloging-in-Publication Data

Names: Davies, Ffion C. W., author. | Bruce, Colin E., author. | Taylor-Robinson, Kate., author.
Title: Emergency care of minor trauma in children / Ffion Davies, Colin E. Bruce, Kate Taylor-Robinson.
Description: Third edition. | Boca Raton : CRC Press, [2017] | Preceded by Emergency care of minor trauma in children / Ffion C.W. Davies, Colin E. Bruce, Kate Taylor-Robinson. London : Hodder Arnold, 2011. | Includes index.
Identifiers: LCCN 2017001548 (print) | LCCN 2017002229 (ebook) | ISBN 9781138048294 (hardback : alk. paper) | ISBN 9781498787710 (pbk. : alk. paper) | ISBN 9781315381312 (Master eBook)
Subjects: | MESH: Emergency Treatment | Adolescent | Child | Infant | Critical Care—methods | Wounds and Injuries—therapy | Handbooks
Classification: LCC RJ370 (print) | LCC RJ370 (ebook) | NLM WS 39 | DDC 618.92/0025—dc23
LC record available at https://lccn.loc.gov/2017001548

Visit the Taylor & Francis Web site at
http://www.taylorandfrancis.com

and the CRC Press Web site at
http://www.crcpress.com

Printed and bound by CPI Group (UK) Ltd, Croydon, CR0 4YY

TABLE OF CONTENTS

We all remember injuring ourselves during our childhood. Minor trauma is a normal part of growing up, and in developed countries the majority of people will have attended an emergency department (ED) with an injury by the age of 18 years. Children are therefore high users of emergency services, and emergency services spend quite a lot of their time seeing children!

This is not a full textbook of minor trauma. The purpose of this handbook is to enable doctors, nurses and emergency nurse practitioners based in hospitals, minor injury units/urgent care or ambulatory centres and general/family practice to manage common minor injuries, know when to ask for help and spot when the 'minor injury' has more significance and is not actually minor.

Although the advice in this book is based on UK practice, the types of minor injuries sustained by children, and the best way of managing them, are similar worldwide. Minor trauma is one of the poorest-researched areas of medicine and the quality of the scientific literature is generally poor, so much of this book is drawn from experience in practice.

A child's minor injury should not be seen in isolation. In fact, the effect of something as simple as being in a plaster cast and missing school to attend follow-up appointments is seen as far from 'minor' by the family, so the term 'minor injury' is a bit of a misnomer. We need to ensure that the take-home advice we give is sensible and practical to the whole family.

As healthcare professionals we also need to consider our approach to the children and treat them with respect and compassion, being aware that the care they receive influences their behaviour and fears the next time they need medical help. Children should be seen in a child-friendly environment, ideally audio-visually separated from adults. This area should be designed for their needs with child-sized equipment, room for play and examination and treatment rooms that are bright and welcoming. It is quite easy to transform an area with brightly coloured paint and posters, and funding is often readily available from local charities. Toys can be used as distraction therapy during painful procedures and for entertainment during periods of observation or waiting. A lot of your medical examination can be conducted through play, rather than a formal examination on a couch. Attention to these aspects really helps you and the child get the job done, in a happy way.

It is also our responsibility to pick up safeguarding issues – in other words suboptimal care or supervision. You can be forgiven for thinking that paediatric-trained colleagues can be obsessed by this, but it is vital that we detect these issues, which are unfortunately common.

Finally, if you would like more help with creating a good emergency service for children, internationally defined *Standards of Care for Children in Emergency Departments* is available from the International Federation of Emergency Medicine at https://www.ifem.cc.

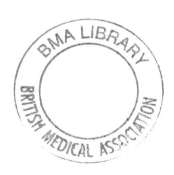

LIST OF VIDEOS

CHAPTER 1

PREVENTION OF INJURY

Injury is a leading cause of death and permanent disability in children and young adults in all countries. Most parents worry about how to let a child explore and learn, yet protect them from accidents. What is an 'accident'? Many injuries in children could be avoided by adequate supervision and common-sense measures, so in a purest sense many are truly 'accidents'. When true neglect to care for a child's safely occurs it is important that we identify it and know what to do (see Chapter 14, Non-accidental Injury).

As health professionals we have a role in educating the families we see and our local community, while striking a balance between advising on injury prevention and encouraging activity and sports for the child's future health. We can be quite influential. A few gentle words of advice at the time of an injury are often remembered. So it is a good opportunity to talk about the patterns of injury that we regularly see when we spot an injury which could have been avoided.

Most injuries to children less than three years of age occur in the home or garden. At this age children develop rapidly, and their carers often underestimate their capabilities. When children become older they attend nurseries or schools, and move further from home for play and other activities. Many incidents leading to injury then occur in schools and sports facilities or in the neighbourhood. As children reach adolescence, injuries occur further from the home or in high-risk places (railway lines, derelict buildings) where bored teenagers seek adventure. There is a strong association between injury rates and social deprivation.

Many organisations exist in developed countries to promote injury prevention and have leaflets and websites with information. In the UK, health visitors assist families with accident prevention. Health professionals should be familiar with advising on simple measures such as:

- Inexpensive safety equipment, e.g. stair gates, fire-guards
- Child-resistant containers for medicines
- Safe storage of household cleaners and garden products
- Safe positioning of hot objects, e.g. cups of tea, kettles, pans, irons

- Safe use of equipment, for example not to put babies in baby bouncers or baby chairs on work surfaces and to always supervise the use of baby walkers
- Safety awareness on roads and railways
- Cycle helmets when riding a bicycle

Worldwide, the most effective way to reduce death and disability has been through compulsory (legal) interventions such as the wearing of seat-belts in cars, fencing around open water, wearing crash helmets when on a bicycle/motorbike/horse, safety locks on the windows of buildings over one storey high and severe speed restrictions in residential areas. Many of these legal interventions came about because we as healthcare professionals raised awareness of the problem, assisting with data collection or noticing local safety hot-spots, and bringing our concerns to local and national level.

CHAPTER 2

PAIN MANAGEMENT

INTRODUCTION

Minor injuries cause pain. Recognition and alleviation of pain should be a priority when treating injuries. This process should ideally start on arrival to your facility and finish with ensuring that adequate analgesia is provided at discharge.

Pain is often under-recognised and under-treated in children. There are several reasons for this. Assessing pain in children can be difficult. For example, children in pain may be quiet and withdrawn, rather than crying. Communication may be difficult with an upset child, and it may be difficult to distinguish pain from other causes of distress (fear, stranger anxiety, etc.). Choosing the right words so that you and the child understand each other means listening or asking what words the family uses, e.g. hurt, sore, poorly. In some cases children may deny pain for fear of the ensuing treatment (particularly needles).

There is often insecurity about dosage of medication in children, which has to be worked out in mg/kg. Some medications are not licensed for use in children, although are commonly used. And there are practical issues such as the psychological and real issues of inserting a cannula for intravenous analgesia.

WHAT ARE WE TREATING?

- *Pain* – This requires analgesia (see below).
- *Fear of the situation* – All efforts should be made to provide a calm, friendly environment. You should explain what you are doing, prepare the child for any procedures and let the parents

stay with the child unless they prefer not to or are particularly distressed.

- *Loss of control* – Children like to be involved in decisions and feel that they are being listened to.
- *Fear of the injury* – Distraction and other cognitive techniques are extremely useful (see below). A little explanation and reassurance goes a long way to allay anxiety.
- *Fear of the treatment* – Unfortunately, some treatments hurt and are frightening in themselves (e.g. sutures). There are lots of things you can do to make procedures less stressful all round; this is covered below.

ASSESSMENT OF PAIN

Pain assessment and treatment now forms an integral part of quality assurance standards for emergency departments in many countries and features in most triage guidelines.

 If there is severe pain, is there a major injury or ischaemia?

Your prior experience of injuries can help in estimating the amount of pain the child is likely to be in. For example a fractured shaft of femur or a burn are more painful than a bump on the head. After that, you will rely on what the child says and how the child behaves.

Clearly, the younger the child, the less they are able to describe how they are feeling, and separating out the distress caused by pain versus distress caused by other factors is tricky. Some children with mild pain can be very upset, due to the stress of the whole situation, the circumstances of the accident, their prior experience of healthcare or because their parents are upset. Having a reassuring environment and staff trained to be comfortable in dealing with distressed children makes a big difference.

Asking a child to rate their pain is difficult; they have little life experience to draw upon and may not clearly remember previous painful episodes, yet we are asking them to make a judgement of whether they are experiencing mild pain or the worst pain they have ever had! Linear analogue scales of 0–10 or comparisons with stairs or a ladder are often too abstract for a child.

Faces scores showing emotions such as those in Table 2.1 are frequently used for self-reporting of pain in children. They have value but cannot be

Table 2.1 Pain assessment tool suitable for children

	No pain	Mild pain	Moderate pain	Severe pain
Faces scale score	(face)	(face)	(face)	(face)
Ladder score	0	1-3	4-6	7-10
Behaviour	Normal activity No ↓ movement Happy	Rubbing affected area Decreased movement Neutral expression Able to play/talk normally	Protective of affected area ↓ movement/quiet Complaining of pain Consolable crying Grimaces when affected part moved/touched	No movement or defensive of affected part Looking frightened Very quiet Restless, unsettled Complaining of lots of pain Inconsolable crying
Injury example	Bump on head	Abrasion Small laceration Sprain ankle/knee # fingers/clavicle Sore throat	Small burn/scald Finger tip injury # forearm/elbow/ankle Appendicitis	Large burn # long bone/dislocation Appendicitis Sickle crisis
Category chosen (tick)				

used in isolation, as they can also be flawed. Children may misunderstand the question because a spectrum of pain can be too difficult a concept. They may point to the happy face because that is how they want to feel or choose the saddest face to reflect how sad they feel.

Taking all of these issues into account, it is clearly better to use a composite score rather than relying on one system. Table 2.1 shows a suggested pain assessment tool recommended by the UK Royal College of Emergency Medicine; the assessor uses the available information to decide what category the pain is. It combines objective and subjective information and staff experience to give an overall score of no, mild, moderate or severe pain.

Once you've treated the pain (see below) you must reassess the child after the medication has had time to work. Failure to reassess and identify inadequate analgesia is, unfortunately, quite common. You should document the new pain score when you reassess.

HOW TO TREAT PAIN

Having assessed the degree of pain, there are a range of ways to treat pain. These include psychological strategies, practical treatments and medication (via various routes). A working knowledge of all the options is useful, so that your treatment is appropriate for the child's age and preference, type of injury and degree of pain.

Psychological strategies

Psychological strategies should be relevant to the age of child, but are useful in all situations. Many children object to practical procedures, even if the procedure is not painful. This generates a lot of anxiety in parents and staff alike. Experienced staff are invaluable when handling distressed children. It is important to be reassuring but sympathetic. Good communication at a level appropriate to the child and good listening skills make a big difference. Looking confident matters, since apprehension is always noticed!

Psychological preparation helps; for example, explain with carefully chosen words, focus on the endpoint, demonstrate on a doll or toy using the right equipment and allow parents to bargain around getting home as soon as possible or receiving rewards.

Next you need to provide distraction during the procedure. Th[...] from infants to teenagers and your unit should have a selection [...] appropriate toys. It is usually relatively easy to obtain toys from [...] and local fundraising. Just be aware of your organisation's antimicrobial policies. Distraction aids include bubbles to blow, murals on walls, books, videos, computer games etc. Smartphones are successful at any age! Music is both soothing and distracting.

It is important to perform procedures swiftly, and not to explain the procedure to the child and then leave them worrying about it while you go and do something else. Try to perform your procedure while allowing the parent contact with their child. Keep the momentum moving forwards and do not allow excessive procrastination or bargaining if the child is trying to avoid the procedure. In some hospitals play specialists are available to calm children waiting to be seen, prepare them for what will happen during the consultation, provide distraction during procedures and give rewards afterwards. There is no hard evidence but in clinical areas where play specialists are employed, staff feel that children are treated with less stress, much quicker and with less recourse to sedation or hospital admission for general anaesthesia. Without play specialists, it is still quite possible to provide the right environment and some basic psychological techniques to achieve the same outcome.

Practical treatments

Injured limbs are usually less painful if elevated (see Chapter 15, Practical Procedures). Fractures are usually less painful if immobilised in splints or a plaster cast. Soft tissue injuries feel better if cooled. Application of an ice pack, avoiding direct contact of ice with skin, can be helpful, although small children dislike ice packs. A lot of the pain from burns comes from air currents, which can be reduced with kitchen cling-wrap if access is still needed, and a proper dressing as soon as possible.

Medication options

There are numerous options for analgesia, with differences between different organisations and different countries. These options are just suggestions. Figure 2.1 describes a practical pain strategy.

 For major injuries, seek senior advice and obtain IV access!

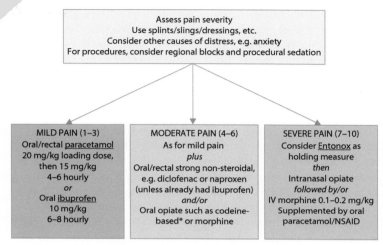

 Figure 2.1 Example of a pain treatment strategy. *In the UK codeine-based drugs are not recommended under the age of 12 years.

Oral medication

Mild pain may be treated with paracetamol (acetaminophen) or non-steroidal anti-inflammatory drugs such as ibuprofen.

Moderate pain may be treated with a combination of both paracetamol and an anti-inflammatory drug. Opioids can be added in, depending on your local guidelines. In the UK codeine-based drugs are not recommended under the age of 12 years. Diclofenac is a stronger anti-inflammatory than ibuprofen.

Severe pain may be treated with oral morphine solution but this takes around 20 minutes to start working.

Intranasal analgesia

Intranasal opiates work more quickly than oral opiates. Intravenous opiates should not be avoided, but in many situations the intranasal opiate will give you 30–60 minutes of good analgesia and anxiolysis, allowing you to get venous access when the child is less stressed. These include intranasal diamorphine 0.1 mg/kg or fentanyl (1.7 mcg/kg) and have an onset of action within 2 minutes, an offset in 30–60 minutes. They are highly effective and have the added benefit of anxiolysis, so they are in widespread use in many countries. They are well tolerated and often avoid needles because by the time dressings or splints have been applied, oral medication has started to work, the child's trust is gained and pain is often under control. If ongoing analgesia is needed, insertion of an IV line is much easier and less traumatic because the initial pain is often under control.

Inhalational analgesia

Thirty per cent nitrous oxide and oxygen (Entonox®) can be provided in cylinders with a face mask or intra-oral delivery system. It depends on the child's cooperation and coordination, and understanding that it is self-activated. For continuous administration of nitrous oxide see the 'Procedural Sedation' section.

Topical anaesthesia

Local anaesthetic creams used for cannulation are not licensed for use on open wounds, but there are gel formulations available for use on wounds such as LAT gel (lignocaine 0.4%, adrenaline 0.1% and tetracaine 0.5%). These are very useful and usually mean that local infiltration of anaesthesia (with a needle) is not needed. Topical preparations can also be used to aid deep cleaning of abrasions. They are mostly licensed for use over the age of 1 year. Do not use on mucous membranes (e.g. near the eyes or mouth). Onset of action is 20–30 minutes and offset 30–60 minutes after removal.

In the case of LAT gel, apply 2 mL to the wound in 1- to 3-year-olds and 3 mL in older children. Then cover with a small square of gauze and overlay a non-occlusive dressing. On removal 20–30 minutes later the skin will appear blanched. Should additional local anaesthesia be needed after testing for pain, only 0.1 mg/kg of lignocaine can be used, due to lignocaine already being present in the LAT gel.

Local infiltration of anaesthesia

Infiltration of local anaesthetic is painful and may not be justified if only one or two sutures are required. Consider LAT gel for wound management, if available. The pain of injection can be reduced by using a narrow bore needle (e.g. a dental needle), by slow injection (see Chapter 15) and probably by buffering and warming the solution.

Regional anaesthesia

Nerve blocks are easy to learn, well tolerated by children and avoid the risks of sedation and respiratory depression. Particularly useful nerve blocks are the femoral or 'three in one' nerve blocks for a fractured femur, the infra-auricular block for removing earrings and digital or metacarpal nerve blocks for fingers (see Chapter 15).

Intravenous (IV) analgesia

IV opiates such as morphine are used when immediate analgesia is required. There should be no hesitation in administering these drugs to children provided care is taken and resuscitation facilities are available. IV fentanyl or propofol should only be used for procedural sedation (see section below).

 Respiratory depression and drowsiness may occur with IV opiates!

Respiratory depression may be avoided by titration, starting with the recommended minimum dose and waiting a few minutes before giving further doses. Naloxone should not be required as an antidote if you titrate opiates, but should be available in your department. Anti-emetics are not usually required in young children.

Intramuscular route (IM)

This route is best avoided as it subjects the child to a needle and holds no advantage over the IV route. Absorption is unpredictable and often slow, making repeated doses (and therefore needles) necessary, and the dosage difficult to calculate. It can be useful for ketamine (see next section), as the child has retrograde amnesia for the injection itself.

PROCEDURAL SEDATION

A wider discussion of the various techniques for procedural sedation is beyond this handbook. Procedural sedation is practiced in many emergency departments worldwide, but it is not suitable for most other urgent care settings, as full resuscitation equipment and skills are needed. It holds benefits for the child (amnesia as well as analgesia) and fills a useful middle ground between minor procedures and distraction (discussed previously) and recourse to general anaesthesia, which helps the family. Many countries and hospitals have guidelines for safe procedural sedation.

Adequate monitoring, trained staff and resuscitation facilities are essential. Do not attempt procedural sedation unless your unit fulfils the basic requirements!

Midazolam is a benzodiazepine which may be given orally, intranasally, rectally or intravenously (IV). Oral midazolam at a dose of 0.5 mg/kg provides mild anxiolysis within 10–15 minutes, but has wide individual variation in effect and can cause hyperactivity. It is most useful in facilitating distraction, such as when removing a foreign body. The oral route is less likely to cause a rapid peak in drug levels than the rectal route and is better tolerated than the intranasal route, which may cause local irritation. Midazolam is not an analgesic. IV midazolam is often combined with an IV opiate for procedures such as fracture or dislocation reduction. The adverse effects of both drugs combined are higher than with a single agent and only experienced doctors should use this combination.

Nitrous oxide 50%, with 50% oxygen administered continuously, provides analgesia, anxiolysis and amnesia. Monitoring and resuscitation facilities are needed. Ketamine is a more effective and safe drug which provides 'dissociative anaesthesia' and has become the preferred option for procedural sedation in the UK and many other countries. Upper respiratory tract symptoms or abnormal airway anatomy (e.g. history of prolonged neonatal ventilation, abnormal face shape) are the main contraindications to the use of ketamine. It may be given IV (ideally) or IM. The IV route allows you to titrate the dose and wears off quicker. A dose of 2.5 mg/kg IM or 1–2 mg/kg IV works within 3 minutes and allows you to perform procedures lasting up to 20 minutes with the child remaining undistressed.

Ketamine may cause hypersalivation which, rarely, may cause laryngospasm. Also, children are at risk of agitation and hallucinations in the 'emergence' phase as the drug wears off, so should therefore be allowed to recover in a quiet room, although still under close nursing observation. Published guidelines also provide useful templates for monitoring, discharge criteria and parental advice post-discharge. IV propofol is also gaining in popularity but its use is not yet mainstream in the UK.

WOUNDS AND SOFT TISSUE INJURIES

Wounds and superficial injuries are common in childhood. Often the child is distressed by the wound itself (and bleeding), the parents will worry about scarring and both parents and staff may be reticent about the procedure of wound repair itself. The use of psychological techniques, an experienced nurse and adequate analgesia will make the procedure more endurable for all (see Chapter 2).

You can avoid most pitfalls related to wound management by stopping to ask yourself – how exactly did this happen? Are there likely to be associated injuries? What lies underneath this wound, anatomically? Is this a simple wound which is suitable for simple repair or do I need expert help? For specific areas, you can refer to the following chapters: face, Chapter 4; hand, Chapter 8; genitalia, Chapter 13.

BASIC HISTORY

Here we will outline some important questions you can ask to take a basic history.

Mechanism of injury

A precise history is needed to alert you to potential problems. For example:

- Underlying injury to tendons/nerves (e.g. wound from something sharp)

- Hidden foreign body (e.g. wound from broken glass)
- Significant head injury (e.g. fall from higher than child's head height)
- Significant blood loss (e.g. wound over blood vessel such as femoral canal)
- Non-accidental injury (e.g. injury in non-mobile child)

By asking What? How? Where?, you will spot important pitfalls!

Time of injury

Wounds over 12 hours old may be better left to heal by secondary intention. If the wound is clean it may be repaired up to 24 hours later, particularly if it is on the face or scalp. You should consider prescribing an antibiotic such as flucloxacillin if suturing an injury after 12 hours.

Tetanus immunisation status

Most children in the UK will be fully vaccinated. Routine immunisations are given at 2, 3 and 4 months old, then again preschool and aged 14–15. This confers lifelong immunity. If an immunisation has been missed, the opportunity should be taken to provide it (if there are departmental arrangements to ensure communication with primary care/community colleagues to avoid duplication). In a non-immunised child this will not provide cover in time for the existing wound, so if the wound is dirty anti-tetanus immunoglobulin should also be given.

Concurrent illness

This is rarely an issue in children and does not affect wound repair. If the child is immunosuppressed or on long-term steroid treatment, follow-up to check wound healing at 5–7 days is advisable. Remember that children with chronic illness may be more needle-phobic.

Consideration of non-accidental injury and accident prevention

The circumstances of the accident need to be given adequate attention (see Chapter 14). However, wounds more often raise concerns about supervision of the child rather than actual deliberate injury. In the UK the health visitor should be notified for all injuries to preschool children. They will identify issues around accident prevention, and may subsequently visit the family at home.

BASIC EXAMINATION

Here is what to look for when taking a wound description.

Site

When writing your notes, always draw diagrams, which are clearer to understand than a written description. Think through the anatomical structures underlying the wound. Is there potential damage to tendons, nerves, blood vessels or the joint capsule? Bleeding can be significant from scalp wounds or from concealed vessel injury, such as the groin. The skin surrounding and distal to the wound should be normal colour and have normal sensation, and distal pulses and capillary refill should be tested and documented.

Test for tendons and nerves where you can. Full strength against resistance should be tested for muscle groups and tendons. Assessment is harder in preverbal children. Where you cannot test, or there is the possibility of deep, serious injury, the wound may need exploration by a surgical colleague. Site also affects wound healing, so bear that in mind when thinking about whether follow-up is needed.

If in doubt, always seek expert advice!

Size

Large wounds may need suturing under general anaesthesia. Calculate the maximum safe dose of local anaesthetic for the child's weight. If this is likely to be exceeded, a general anaesthetic may be needed, if there is not a suitable alternative regional block (see Chapter 15). Other than anaesthetic issues, size in itself does not affect the choice of options for closure.

Depth

Depth affects the likelihood of damage to underlying structures, and your options for closure (see the section 'General principles of wound repair'). The most innocent-looking wound on the surface can conceal serious complications, if it is a stab wound or a puncture wound. Deep wounds may need two layers of suture – an inner, absorbable layer as well as the skin sutures.

Seek senior advice immediately for stab wounds! Treat Airway, Breathing, Circulation, Disability, before focussing on the wound.

FACTORS INVOLVED IN HEALING

Wounds generally heal better in children than adults. Wound healing is very individual, and in growing children the appearance of the scar can change for up to 2 years. Therefore, avoid being either very positive or very negative when asked about future appearance.

Children with pigmented skin may have hypopigmentation of the affected area, either for a year or so or long-term. Those of Afro-Caribbean origin may develop keloid scars. Sun sensitivity may be a problem for 6 to 12 months in any race, so recommend protective creams. Many wounds itch when healing, and simple moisturisers (particularly those used for treating eczema) are useful.

Site of injury

Healing is quickest in wounds on the face, mouth and scalp, due to the richness of the blood supply, and takes longest in the lower body. The tension across a wound is important, and is a major factor in your choice of closure techniques (see the section 'General principles of wound repair'). Delayed healing and/or scarring are most likely when wounds are under tension. It is worth considering splintage to help healing in mobile areas, for example knuckle, knee or heel wounds. There are lines of natural tension in the body. These are called Langer's lines (Figures 3.1 and 3.2).

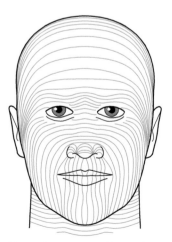

 Figure 3.1 Langer's lines of the face.

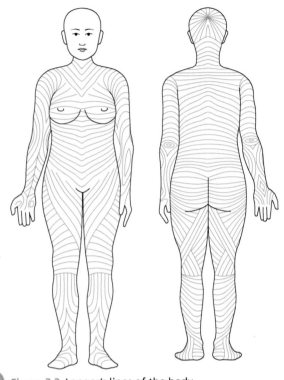

Figure 3.2 Langer's lines of the body.

If a wound is aligned with these lines, healing occurs quicker and is less likely to produce a scar than wounds which cross the lines.

Infection risk

Infection is more likely in dirty areas of the body, e.g. sole of the foot, and obviously, more likely in dirty wounds. Organic material is far more likely to cause infection than inorganic material. Substances such as soil carry a high bacterial load. Also, bacteria multiply in a logarithmic fashion, so the longer a wound remains dirty, the higher the risk. Infection risk is lower in areas with a good blood supply. The more distal the wound (from the head), the greater the likelihood of infection. The more open a wound, the easier it is for infection to drain. This means that puncture wounds are at high risk of infection, despite looking benign (see section 'Specific wounds and areas'). Lastly, wound infection may be a sign of a foreign body. See the section 'Foreign bodies' for a discussion of this.

Puncture wounds are at high risk of infection!

Wound edges

Wounds that heal best and scar least have healthy, straight edges. Crush injuries are more likely to produce swelling and ragged edges which are difficult to oppose, causing delayed healing and scarring. They may also damage the skin, causing haematoma formation and jeopardising viability. Shaved edges (sometimes with skin loss) are likely to heal with a visible scar. If wound edges look severely damaged, it is often worth waiting a few days to judge viability in children, rather than immediately debriding the edges; children can recover well. If you are unsure, ask a more experienced doctor.

GENERAL PRINCIPLES OF WOUND MANAGEMENT

Abrasions

Abrasions may be of variable depth, and can be described and treated in a similar way to burns. At initial presentation every attempt must be made to get the wound as clean as possible, using local anaesthesia if needed. In children, abrasions may be contaminated with road tar, which has the potential to cause 'tattooing'.

If the wound is inadequately cleaned, dirt particles become ingrained and cause permanent disfigurement. Forceps, surgical brushes or needles may be used to clear wounds of debris. If the surface area to be cleaned is so large that the dose of local anaesthetic may be exceeded, general anaesthesia may be necessary. If a little dirt remains, this may work its way out over the next few days and dressings and creams such as those used to deslough chronic ulcers may be helpful. Follow-up in 4–5 days' time is necessary in this situation.

Cleaning and irrigation of wounds

All wounds should be considered dirty to an extent, but those contaminated with organic material are particularly at risk of infection. Good wound toilet, with adequate dilution of the bacterial load with copious water, is far more important than relying on prophylactic antibiotics. See Chapter 15 for how to irrigate a wound. There is little evidence for antiseptic solutions being any better than water at preventing infections, and they sting more.

Exploration of wounds

Exploration of a wound should be considered when a foreign body or damage to underlying structures is suspected. However, it often requires several injections to create an anaesthetic field, and some children may not understand or tolerate this, or in fact tolerate prolonged periods of wound exploration. Consider this before you start. Also consider how much local anaesthetic you are likely to need. If this exceeds the safe total dose for the child's weight, the child will need a regional or general anaesthetic. If you think you will need more experienced help, it is better to get this at the outset than have a child waiting halfway through a procedure, getting anxious. Lastly, never extend a wound's size without seeking advice first.

Foreign bodies

See also Chapter 12. Foreign bodies such as grit and oil may cause tattooing if left (see 'Abrasions', above). If there is a foreign body within the wound and this is not suspected or detected, the wound is likely to become infected, heal slowly or break down again.

Always consider the potential presence of a foreign body in any infected wound!

Always request a soft tissue X-ray if an injury has been caused by glass!

Most types of glass are radio-opaque (see Chapter 12, Figure 12.1). Fragments are notoriously difficult to spot with the naked eye, and may lie deep. If glass has been removed from a wound, a follow-up X-ray must be performed to check it is all gone. Other types of foreign body are not radio-opaque, including plant material such as wood. However, these can often be clearly demonstrated by ultrasound.

GENERAL PRINCIPLES OF WOUND REPAIR

See Chapter 15 (Practical Procedures) for application of adhesive strips and glue, anaesthesia (local infiltration and regional blocks) and insertion of sutures.

Primary repair or not?

Wounds over 12 hours old (24 hours for facial or scalp wounds), bites and those which are contaminated, contused or devitalised are more likely to become infected. In these cases you will often be best advised to leave the wound unclosed, with a dressing over the top. It will heal by 'secondary intention'. This means healing by granulation from the bottom up and eventual re-epithelialisation over the top. In such wounds, sutures act as an additional foreign body and increase the risk of infection; opposition of the wound edges (either by sutures or adhesive strips) makes the underlying wound anaerobic and more prone to infection. The outcome can be a lot more protracted, with worse scarring, than if the wound had been left open. To speed this process up, splintage can be very useful (e.g. of a knee or elbow, or Achilles tendon area).

In certain circumstances delayed primary closure after 4–5 days is appropriate. This means not attempting any closure until that time, to minimise the risk of infection. If you are thinking of leaving a wound to heal by secondary intention, seek advice about the option of delayed closure. Wounds with skin loss should also usually be allowed to heal by secondary intention, rather than creating tension by trying to achieve primary closure. Wounds with skin loss of less than a squared centimetre tend to do well, and even larger areas will often heal in children, without recourse to skin grafting.

If in doubt, always seek expert advice!

Choice of technique for wound closure

While interrupted sutures are what we often do, and are often perceived as the gold standard in wound repair, in fact the cosmetic result is as good with adhesive strips or glue, provided there is no tension on the wound. So in practice, judge if you need sutures to hold the wound edges together. If the edged are easily opposed, adhesive strips or glue usually suffice. Factors such as Langer's lines (see 'Factors involved in healing', above) are more important than depth. However, if sutures are indicated, do not avoid sutures simply because of the practical difficulties of suturing children. A good cosmetic result is paramount.

Tissue glue has excellent cosmetic results. It needs to be applied properly (see Chapter 15) and can sting as it is applied. It both rubs off and dissolves after about 2 weeks. Adhesive strips are often known by parents as 'butterfly stitches' and are easy to apply. They are easy to remove after a few days, especially if wetted. Glue tolerates a few splashes or occasional immersion in water better than adhesive strips. Staples are sometimes used, but patients and parents find them off-putting, and removal can be tricky. In mobile areas of the body or in fidgety children, glue with overlaid adhesive strips can be a useful technique.

AFTERCARE

Dressings and bandages

There is a lot of debate but not much scientific evidence for 'the right dressing'. There is often less focus on how to do 'the right bandage' but in practical terms, for children this is crucial. Many bandages do not last much longer than the child leaving your treatment area, then the dressing will fall off too. For tips on longevity see Chapter 15.

The purpose of a dressing is to prevent additional contamination of the wound and to provide a barrier to air currents and friction against clothing, etc. Wounds that are oozing (blood or serous fluid) must be dressed with a non-stick dressing, so that changing the dressing in the next day or two does not hurt or disturb the wound too much. Paraffin impregnated gauze is a suitable dressing.

After the first 24–72 hours, silicon-based dressings are particularly useful, but other non-stick dressings can be used. It is best to leave the wound undisturbed for a few days, unless it is at high risk of infection. Unfortunately, despite the tricks of the trade, children often pull dressings off, or get them wet or dirty, necessitating more frequent dressing changes. A more detailed discussion of wound dressing is too large a topic to be covered in this book, and there is a great deal of variation, depending on local circumstances.

Prophylactic antibiotics

Good wound cleaning (see 'Cleaning and irrigation of wounds', above) is more important than antibiotic treatment. Antibiotics are only necessary if there is a high risk of infection. This means wounds contaminated with organic material, or bites. An anti-staphylococcal and anti-streptococcal agent such as flucloxacillin is appropriate. Cover for Gram-negative organisms is only needed for certain animal bites (see Chapter 11, Bites, Stings and Allergic Reactions), oral or perineal wounds or those sustained in muddy areas or water.

Tetanus prophylaxis

See 'Basic history' section at the beginning of this chapter.

Immobilisation

If a wound is over a mobile area such as a joint, for example, a large wound over the knee, wound healing is often speeded up considerably, and scarring reduced, if the part is immobilised with a splint or small plaster of Paris for a week or two. In this short period of time, stiffness is not really an issue with children, compared with adults.

Suture removal

If sutures are left in too long there is an increased risk of infection, and of suture marks being visible on the skin permanently. Children heal much quicker than adults, so sutures can usually be removed on day 4 on the face, and day 5 on other areas, unless under tension. The wound can always be supported by adhesive strips for a few days after sutures are removed.

COMMON COMPLICATIONS

Infection

Infection is more likely in wounds that are dirty or contain a foreign body, those with contused or crushed skin, puncture wounds or those with a delay in treatment or cleaning. If a wound becomes infected, consider the presence of a foreign body. It may sometimes be difficult to tell if a wound is infected but signs include slow healing, ongoing oozing, surrounding erythema, smell and pain. Spreading cellulitis, lymphangitis or systemic upset are indications for intravenous antibiotics.

Wound swabs do not yield useful microbiological results for 2–3 days, so the decision to treat is usually from clinical experience. Treat with an antibiotic such as flucloxacillin, but also immobilise the wound or discourage use of the limb, elevate it if possible and remove sutures if present.

 Infected wounds should be reviewed after 2–5 days!

Dehiscence

If dehiscence occurs, seek surgical advice. Dehiscence almost always means that there is wound infection (unless there has been clear disturbance of the wound).

SPECIFIC WOUNDS AND AREAS

Puncture wounds

Innocent-looking puncture wounds are a minefield to the unwary. Firstly, they may be much deeper than initially suspected, and a thorough clinical examination of underlying structures should be undertaken. Secondly, bacteria are injected deep into tissues. The smaller the wound, the more likely it is to become infected because the overlying skin edges are opposed. Consider antibiotic prophylaxis, unless you can get the nozzle of a syringe into the puncture wound, for gentle irrigation (see Chapter 15).

Needlestick injuries

Hospitals often have a needlestick policy. Children may sustain such injuries when they find discarded needles in areas frequented by drug misusers. If you have no local policy, advise parents that the risk of any blood-borne infection is low, but is higher for hepatitis B than HIV. Seek specialist advice.

Plantar wounds of the foot

These wounds are notorious for their propensity to develop infection, particularly *Pseudomonas aeruginosa*, often after a delay of several days to a few weeks. Patients should be advised to return if foot pain increases, and appropriate specialist advice sought if this occurs. An antibiotic such as ciprofloxacin is often prescribed prophylactically. Find out if you have a local policy.

HAEMATOMAS AND CONTUSIONS

A haematoma is a large bruise with a large collection of blood. A contusion just means bruising. Bruising is common in children, and normally affects the lower limbs. Bruising is less common on the trunk or face or behind the ears. If you see bruising in these areas, or see many bruises, ask how they happened (see Chapter 14, Non-accidental Injury). If there are multiple bruises, consider checking the child's platelet count and a clotting screen. The age of a bruise is more difficult to determine than is commonly thought, so you should never comment on the age of a bruise.

 Always assess whether bruising is compatible with the history given, and refer for a second opinion if unsure.

Following blunt injury, a significant amount of bleeding may go on underneath the skin surface and may not be apparent for some days. It will usually come out distal to the actual site of injury, due to gravity. Children are less prone to residual stiffness of the affected muscles than adults, because they heal quicker and are more determined to mobilise early.

Simple initial management of contused areas involves elevation of the affected part if possible and the application of ice packs (avoiding direct contact of the ice on the skin) at regular intervals for the first few hours, if the child will accept this. Early mobilisation will help the blood dissolve. While this is rarely a problem in small children, teenagers may need some encouragement!

SPRAINS

A sprain is a soft tissue injury such as tearing of a ligament. Children have stretchy tissues so are less prone to sprains than adults, and generally recover much quicker. This means you should be careful in diagnosing a simple sprain in toddlers and young children, since an underlying fracture is more likely. Refer to the following chapters for specific sprains: neck, Chapter 5; knee and ankle, Chapter 9.

The management of a sprain is similar to a contusion (see the previous section). Early mobilisation should be encouraged. Most emergency departments have advice sheets for common sprains such as the ankle, shoulder or knee. The mnemonic 'RICE' is often used: rest, ice, compression and elevation. However, most children are reluctant to rest or elevate their limb for very long, and there is little evidence that more than 24 hours of rest is beneficial. Ice packs can be applied a few times in the first 12 hours. Direct contact of ice with skin should be avoided, and packets of frozen vegetables wrapped in a tea towel are a practical choice for most households! A compression bandage may help reduce swelling but does not provide support or improve healing.

COMPARTMENT SYNDROME

In certain areas of the body, particularly the forearm and lower leg, the muscles are grouped together in compartments, separated by fascia. Following injury, swelling occurs, and can be accommodated up to a point. Thereafter, the pressure inside the compartment rises, the blood supply via the arterioles becomes jeopardised and the muscles become ischaemic. A vicious cycle develops, which can result in necrosis, rhabdomyolysis, contractures and even loss of limb. This is much less common in children than adults, and is usually associated with limb fractures in teenagers.

Pulses often remain present until late on in the process. Early symptoms are pain and paraesthesia. Passive stretching of the muscles is extremely painful and the limb may appear swollen. If in doubt, the pressure inside the compartment can be measured using a needle and transducer (pressures above 30 mmHg are worrying). Urgently opening up the whole compartment with a fasciotomy under general anaesthesia may be needed.

An urgent surgical opinion is necessary for suspected compartment syndrome!

DEGLOVING INJURIES

Degloving injuries occur when the skin and its blood supply are avulsed. This occurs with a blunt, shearing mechanism of injury and may not be obvious in the early stages, particularly if no laceration of the skin has occurred. Areas prone to this kind of injury are the scalp, lower leg and foot. A typical mechanism of injury would be a car wheel running over the leg. On examination, the skin is often contused and may be mobile. Swelling and/or an underlying fracture need not necessarily be present. Initial management consists of elevation of the limb or compression for a scalp laceration. A plastic surgeon must be involved, often jointly with an orthopaedic surgeon, since microsurgery, external fixation of fractures, fasciotomy or skin grafting may be necessary.

It may be very difficult to spot a degloving injury, so always think about the mechanism of the injury!

SKIN ABSCESSES

An abscess is a contained infection that may be caused by a breach of the skin, an infected hair follicle or often for no obvious reason. They are relatively uncommon in children, and the presence of a foreign body should be considered. A common abscess in children is a paronychia (see Chapter 8).

Once pus has collected, it cannot be treated successfully with antibiotics, but requires incision and drainage. The abscess may be quite deep seated and require general anaesthesia to achieve enough analgesia to allow full evacuation of its contents. Axillary, perianal and facial abscesses should be referred to a surgeon. For straightforward abscesses, incision and drainage can be performed in the emergency department. This is best achieved with infiltration of local anaesthesia, and a large incision made to allow the pus out and to continue to drain. A non-adhesive dressing should be applied and the patient reviewed by their general practitioner.

HEAD AND FACIAL INJURIES

INTRODUCTION

Head injury is a very common presentation to the emergency department (ED). Head injury is so common in childhood (particularly small toddlers falling over) that parents generally only seek medical help if there is a wound, or if the child was either knocked out or became nauseous or drowsy. Fewer than 1% of children brought to the ED in developed nations will have a positive CT scan, so you can see that the vast majority of children are rapidly discharged home after a brief, clinical examination. The challenge is to spot the child who may have an intracranial bleed, and require neurosurgery or admission for observation. The way to do this is to recognise the importance of the mechanism of injury and the child's behaviour since the event.

Serious head injury is one of the most common causes of death in children.

Most seriously injured children are apparent from the mechanism of injury, and their symptoms and signs (see the next section). Sadly, a small number of infants die each year from non-accidental head injury. For the purposes of this book, a minor head injury is defined as one where the Glasgow coma score (GCS) is *normal*, i.e. the child is alert and orientated.

ASSESSMENT OF HEAD INJURIES

Mechanism of injury

In any age group, injury severity correlates with the distance fallen. Any child falling from higher than their head height must be regarded as high risk. In contrast, toddlers who trip over are low risk. Falling down stairs is medium risk. Infants and toddlers often fall head-first because the head is large compared with the rest of the body.

Non-mobile infants may fall from a height such as parents' arms, a bed or nappy-changing table or a baby chair put on a work surface. Skull fractures are relatively common in these cases. In any non-mobile infant, listen hard to the history. A depressed skull fracture will tend to be caused by something with a small surface area striking the head, such as a golf club, or corner of a table or step. If the baby is said to have rolled off a surface check that the baby is developmentally capable of doing this by playing with them (see Chapter 14, Non-accidental Injury).

 Always consider non-accidental injury in non-mobile infants!

Beware in older children that the true story may be concealed (for example a teenager who does not want to confess what was going on) and it is possible to miss a significant injury unless you stop to consider this.

Symptoms

When you take the history, you must ask directly about the following symptoms: loss of consciousness (beware different phrases for this such as 'knocked out' or appearances such as 'floppy', 'not there', etc.), memory of events during and pre- and post-injury, headache, confusion at any time, agitation or drowsiness, a seizure post-injury and vomiting.

A minor head injury in some toddlers can trigger a 'breath-holding attack', which must be distinguished from loss of consciousness as a result of brain injury. The diagnosis is based on a careful history of a brief interval of consciousness and fright, before apnoea, and sometimes unconsciousness, which may last seconds or minutes. More severe cases will suffer a reflex anoxic seizure. The child recovers back to normal within a minute or so. There may have been previous similar but milder reactions, such as after immunisations. Though frightening, it is an entirely benign phenomenon.

Examination

In any head-injured child, before you start assessment consider if you need to be also examining for cervical spine injury (see Chapter 5), depending on the mechanism of injury. In a child who is alert, your examination needs to include the child's behaviour, examination of the scalp and a formal calculation of the GCS (Table 4.1). A GCS below 15 (normal) means that this is not a minor head injury, and is outside the scope of this book.

 Consider an associated C spine injury!

Measuring the GCS can be a bit tricky in a small child. There are different versions of paediatric coma scores in use, some of which have 14 as the maximum score, so it is best to use the adult score but apply some

 Table 4.1 Glasgow coma scale

Glasgow coma scale		Score
Eyes open	Spontaneously	4
	To speech	3
	To pain	2
	None	1
Best verbal response	Orientated	5
	Conversation disorganized	4
	Inappropriate words	3
	Incomprehensible sound	2
	None	1
Best motor response	Obeys commands, normal spontaneous	6
	Localizes to painful stimulus	5
	Flexes to pain	4
	Abnormal flexor posturing	3
	Abnormal extensor posturing	2
	None	1

common sense. It is useful to describe the child's behaviour. For example, do they interact with the people and environment around them? Are they settled or agitated or drowsy? Assessing the GCS takes practise; keep a copy with you (or look at the ambulance sheet, chart on a wall or an observations/vital signs nursing chart) and keep practising!

If the GCS is less than 15 at any time beyond the first few minutes post-injury, this may not be a minor head injury!

After assessing the GCS, you need to examine the pupils and the scalp. In a fully conscious child, if you see asymmetry of the pupils it is highly unlikely to be due to the head injury (asymmetry implies rapid deterioration due to raised intracranial pressure, which is a late sign, and follows a stage of drowsiness or confusion).

Scalp signs may include lacerations or haematomas. Small, firm haematomas are generally benign, even if quite prominent. Larger, 'boggy' haematomas are highly indicative of underlying fracture, particularly in the under ones. A skull fracture is likely if the haematoma measures more than 5 cm in diameter, or is over the parietal or occipital bone. In a non-walking infant, if there is visible bruising on the face or scalp, non-accidental injury must be considered.

Conventionally we are taught to examine for a base of skull fracture by checking for Battle's sign (bruising behind the ears) and 'panda eyes' (bruising around the eyes). In reality, base of skull fractures are rare in children unless there is a major head injury, and these signs take a few hours to develop. Equally, fundoscopy is largely pointless. By the time the fundi show signs of papilloedema, the child will not have a normal GCS or be behaving normally.

MANAGEMENT OF HEAD INJURIES

Local policies will, for the large part, determine your management. By the time children have arrived in the ED, been observed in the play area while waiting to be seen, then undergone a simple clinical assessment, the vast majority are clearly well enough to be sent home with advice.

The role of X-rays and CT

In children there is a relatively weak correlation between skull fracture and intracranial bleeding, so skull X-rays have no real role if there is access to a CT scanner and there is any cause for concern by history or examination.

In the UK there are national guidelines to help you decide if the child needs a CT head scan. These are derived from the three main decision rules for head injury in children (CHALICE, CATCH and PECARN).

https://www.nice.org.uk/guidance/Cg176

The trickiest decision is usually around a child who has vomited but is otherwise well. Note that in some cases, the head injury is very minor and vomiting is a symptom of new-onset gastroenteritis or viral illness. In the prodrome of these illnesses the child may be feeling unwell and a little off balance, so head injury is more common. If the mechanism of injury sounds very minor and particularly if the time interval between injury and vomiting is a few hours, examine the child for any signs of medical illness and check if they have had recent contact with gastroenteritis cases. Vomiting after head injury usually happens within half an hour. Vomiting once or twice is fairly common, as is the child wanting to sleep for a short period. Vomiting or drowsiness beyond this point means the child needs a head CT scan. If you are unsure, seek senior advice. The radiation of a CT scan is often avoided by allowing a period of observation of up to 8 hours. This is reasonable management if the mechanism of injury was low risk and the child has a GCS of 15.

With modern scanners the child only needs to stay still for 20 seconds or so. The scan is usually possible if the parent is allowed to stay with them, and with a little persuasion and comforting. Failing this, the child's head can be kept still in soft foam or a vacuum mattress. Occasionally general anaesthesia will be needed in order to get an adequate image.

Consult an anaesthetist or senior ED doctor for advice if the child will not stay still for a CT scan!

If the CT scan is positive for acute injury, in most centres the case would be automatically discussed with a neurosurgeon. On the whole, intracranial haematomas are much less common in children than adults. If a subdural haemorrhage is seen in a younger child or infant, always consider non-accidental injury as a possible cause (see Chapter 14, Non-accidental Injury).

Discharge instructions

Children must be watched by a competent adult for the next few hours, and brought back to the ED if they become drowsy, vomit more than once or if the carer is worried that they are not behaving as they normally do. For infants, criteria for returning should be kept broad, and include poor feeding, drowsiness or persistent crying. Children should be allowed to sleep if they want to, but only for as long as is normal for them. You may need to admit a child to hospital for observation if the injury occurred in the evening and it is the child's bedtime.

Parents of older children and teenagers should be advised that headache is a common symptom post–head injury, and may continue for a week or two. They should only be concerned if it is severe, unresponsive to analgesia or associated with drowsiness, change in behaviour, vomiting or confusion. Other symptoms such as dizziness, poor concentration and memory, blurred vision and tiredness are also very common and can be explained to parents using the word 'concussion'. If a child was knocked out for a few seconds, or was a bit dazed and concussed after the injury, they should avoid contact sports for the next 2 weeks in order to avoid 'second impact syndrome' or long-term cognitive problems.

SCALP LACERATIONS

The scalp has an excellent blood supply so small wounds can bleed a lot, causing alarm. Most wounds will have stopped bleeding within 10 minutes, but rarely, bleeding can be hard to control. If a pressure bandage wrapped around the head does not achieve haemostasis, the wound needs prompt insertion of some sutures through all the layers, to tamponade the bleeding. It is useful if you use lidocaine local anaesthetic with added adrenaline for this situation. The adrenaline causes vasospasm and helps you see the field of operation. For wound closure options and techniques, see Chapters 3 and 15.

 STOP Read the following sections in conjunction with Chapter 3, Wounds and Soft Tissue Injuries, and Chapter 15, Practical Procedures.

FACIAL LACERATIONS

Facial lacerations may bleed profusely. This rich blood supply means that wounds generally heal quickly, and infection is unusual, even in bites.

However, facial scars are noticed easily. Senior ED staff, orofaciomaxillary (OFM) and plastic surgeons are always happy to be referred difficult facial wounds in children. Suturing of faces is traumatic for most children, and it may be necessary to use procedural sedation (see Chapter 2) or to refer for repair under general anaesthesia. Forehead wounds may bruise in the coming days, and bruising tracks down to the periorbital area. It is worth warning parents about this innocent complication.

If you lack confidence in ensuring a cosmetic repair for difficult areas, seek help!

Eyelid wounds

Eyelid wounds need perfect repair under magnification, so refer to ophthalmology.

Any wound involving the eyelid should be referred to an ophthalmologist!

Eyebrow wounds

Wounds involving the eyebrow require perfect anatomical repair with sutures, in order to avoid a 'step' in the line of the eyebrow, which has very visible cosmetic consequences. Refer to a specialist if you are not confident. Even with accurate initial repair, a step can develop later as the child grows, so parents should be warned about this.

EYE INJURIES

You should be familiar with the use of a slit lamp, and be able to test visual acuity. A modified Snellen chart, using pictures, is available for younger children. Topical anaesthetic drops, e.g. benoxinate and proxymetacaine, are often necessary to facilitate thorough examination, and are effective almost instantly. Duration of action is usually 20–60 minutes. Many painful eye injuries cause blepharospasm and spasm of the ciliary apparatus. Administration of mydriatic drops to dilate the pupil, e.g. cyclopentolate, can relieve this but are best avoided in young children since they may cause systemic anticholinergic effects. For any breach of the corneal surface, topical antibiotics, e.g. chloramphenicol, should be prescribed for prevention of secondary infection until the patient is asymptomatic. Ointment can be administered twice daily whereas drops require application every 3 hours.

Thus, although ointment blurs vision, it is often easier to administer in children. Photophobia is commonly present, and a feeling of direct pressure can be comforting, so an eye patch may be offered to older children. Patients often request anaesthetic drops to take home, because of the instant relief of symptoms, but this is not advisable because of the risk of secondary injury.

 Visual acuity must always be documented for eye injuries!

Corneal abrasions

Corneal abrasions are caused by the eye being scratched, e.g. by a zip or twig. Babies can sustain corneal abrasions accidentally from their mothers. It is therefore valuable to look for an abrasion if presented with a persistently crying baby. Diagnosis may prevent a series of other investigations! Corneal abrasions tend to be very painful, or may present with a foreign body sensation. Photophobia, watering and injection of the conjunctiva are usually present.

Abrasions are easier to see with fluorescein (orange) staining under a blue light. It is not necessary for a child to cooperate with slit lamp examination; shining the blue or green light of an ophthalmoscope from a distance is less threatening. Cover the eye with a patch and prescribe an antibiotic ointment to prevent secondary infection. Abrasions smaller than the size of the pupil, and not crossing the pupil, do not require follow-up.

Corneal foreign bodies

A small foreign body may enter the eye while working with tools, or simply when carried by the wind. Foreign body detection often requires a slit lamp for magnification. Anaesthetic drops may be needed. If it is not visible on direct view, use a cotton wool bud, with the patient looking downwards, to evert the upper eyelid in case the foreign body is trapped underneath. At this point, if there is still none visible, an abrasion is the most likely finding (see previous section) or often an allergic reaction to a foreign body that has now washed out in the tears (particularly if the foreign body was organic). To remove a foreign body, see Chapter 15. After removal, apply a patch, prescribe antibiotic ointment (see previous section) and arrange follow-up.

Hyphaema

A hyphaema occurs when the eye is struck, and bleeding occurs into the anterior chamber. There is photophobia and a fluid level may be visible in front of the iris, but it may require a slit lamp for detection. Hospital admission may be required. Refer to an ophthalmologist immediately.

Penetrating injuries of the globe

If a sharp object has injured the eye and you examine it using fluorescein (see 'Corneal abrasions', above) you must be sure that penetration of the globe has not occurred. If there is an obvious tear in the cornea or vitreous extrusion, or signs such as an abnormal pupil shape or reaction or decreased acuity, refer immediately to an ophthalmologist because there is a high risk of infection and loss of sight.

 All penetrating injuries must be referred to an ophthalmologist immediately!

Chemical injuries

Children commonly get liquids in their eyes, e.g. household cleaning fluids. Alkaline injuries are more serious than acid splashes, so use litmus paper to see which type of chemical was involved – if the liquid has been brought in with the family, you can test it to avoid testing the eye. Alkalis permeate between cell membranes, causing deep-seated damage. Deceptively, they may be less painful than acids initially. When acid hits the eye, injuries are usually superficial because acids cause coagulation of the surface tissues, thus forming a protective barrier to further damage.

 Alkaline injuries are much more serious than acid injuries!

Alkalis are found in household cleaning products, and may be highly concentrated in substances such as oven cleaner, drain deblocker or liquid dishwasher or laundry capsules. In the UK the National Poisons Information Service online service is able to identify the pH of most commercially available products.

 http://www.toxbase.org

If the fluid is acidic then irrigation using 500 mL of saline solution, via an IV giving set, should suffice. Anaesthetic drops may be needed before you start. No follow-up is necessary unless the child remains symptomatic. If the fluid is alkaline, irrigate immediately and for much longer with larger volumes. If symptoms return over the next hour, seek advice from an ophthalmologist, as the child may need hospital admission for constant irrigation.

Litmus paper is not useful for monitoring response to irrigation! Rely on symptoms.

INJURIES OF THE EAR

The pinna

Wounds through to the cartilage should be referred to OFM or ENT surgeons. A blow to the pinna may cause a haematoma. If this becomes tense, necrosis of the inner cartilage may occur, causing lifelong deformity ('cauliflower ears'). If tense, consult an ENT surgeon for drainage; if not, apply a pressure bandage using a gauze pack and a 'turban' bandage, and arrange review the following day.

The tympanic membrane

This may perforate following a blow to the side of the head, but more typically following foreign body insertion, particularly cotton wool buds (see Chapter 12). Examination may be difficult because of pain. Spontaneous healing usually occurs, but the child should avoid swimming and should be examined by their general practitioner after 3–4 weeks to ensure healing has occurred.

NASAL INJURIES

Nasal fractures

A direct blow to the nose may result in fracture. This is unlikely in children under 7 years because the nasal bone is not calcified. Many parents bring babies and toddlers who have fallen forwards and have a bleeding nose; in these cases you can be very reassuring. Record displacement of the nose, and always document presence or absence of a septal haematoma, which looks like a dark, bulging mass. If a septal haematoma is present, a similar process as happens in the pinna can occur, resulting in a 'saddle nose' deformity. Refer to an ENT specialist immediately for drainage.

Always examine specifically for a septal haematoma!

Nasal fractures are associated with swelling, bony tenderness and sometimes deformity. If you think that there is a nasal fracture, it is not necessary to X-ray for nasal fractures, as the management is symptomatic and/or cosmetic. Advise the patient that the swelling will increase over the next few days and they may develop 'black eyes'. The only treatment is to apply ice packs in the first few hours. Find out your local arrangements for follow-up in an outpatient ENT clinic around 10 days' time. The purpose of follow-up is for consideration of manipulation of the fracture if there is deformity or nasal obstruction. This is impossible to assess in the first few days, hence the delay.

Epistaxis

As just described, nosebleeds may happen with trauma, and are mainly harmless. Spontaneous epistaxis is also common in childhood, usually caused by nose-picking. This causes staphylococcal infection in the anterior nose and scabs. When picked they bleed. If simple pressure does not work (after 30 minutes) then cautery may occasionally be necessary. On discharge it is worth a course of topical antibiotics to get rid of the underlying infection. Recurrent, spontaneous nosebleeds, or protracted bleeding, should prompt you to consider a coagulation disorder or a low platelet count.

ORAL INJURIES

Injuries of the mouth area are common. Fortunately they heal well, but there are a few pitfalls that we will discuss next.

Lacerations crossing the vermillion border of the lip

Wounds crossing the vermillion border of the lip require perfect anatomical repair with sutures, to avoid a 'step' in the line of the lip border, which has greater cosmetic consequences for this complication than for most scars. Despite accurate initial repair, a step may develop later, as the child grows. Parents should be warned about this.

 Wounds crossing the vermillion border require expert repair!

'Through and through' lacerations of the lip

This means that the wound extends from the inside of the mouth to the skin outside, and is usually caused by the teeth. Careful repair with sutures is necessary to avoid cosmetic deformity, accumulation of food in the tract or formation of a sinus. A layered repair may be necessary; do not attempt this yourself unless you have the necessary skills.

Torn frenulum

The frenulum attaches the upper lip to the gum, between the two first incisors. It contains a small artery, which bleeds profusely initially, then usually goes into spasm and stops, particularly if cold compresses and pressure are applied. Suturing is rarely necessary. It is caused by a direct blow to the upper lip. This is commonly due to a toddler falling face first onto a table, a swing swinging backwards into a child, etc. Check the history for a clear account of a direct blow to the upper lip, and ensure the story is told in a natural, plausible manner, remembering to consider inflicted injury (see Chapter 14).

 Check the history!

Wounds of the buccal cavity

Most wounds of the buccal cavity heal quickly by themselves. Sutures are only necessary if they are gaping, or if a piece of tissue will interfere with chewing. Use absorbable materials if sutures are necessary. For this, procedural sedation or general anaesthesia is often needed. Advise soft foods for a few days. Broad-spectrum antibiotics, e.g. co-amoxyclavulanic acid, are frequently prescribed. Warn the parents that the wound will have yellow slough over the next couple of days.

Lacerations of the tongue

The same principles apply as for wounds of the buccal cavity (see the previous section).

Penetrating intra-oral injuries

This type of injury commonly occurs if a child trips while holding something in their mouth. It is important to recognise if the object may have penetrated through the palate. A graze to the hard palate is common. If you see a soft plate wound, it may be hiding a significant injury, which can progress to a retropharyngeal abscess and mediastinitis. If in doubt, request a lateral soft tissue X-ray of the neck and refer to an ENT specialist.

 Failure to recognise perforation of the palate may result in severe illness and even death!

DENTAL INJURIES

The most important consideration in dental injuries is whether the tooth is a primary (deciduous) or permanent tooth. In general, injuries to primary teeth can be reviewed by a dentist the following day.

Avulsion of a tooth

When a permanent tooth is avulsed, the root starts to die within half an hour, so that reimplantation rapidly becomes unsuccessful, or if the tooth reattaches it may become discoloured. Reimplantation needs to happen as soon as possible, and the chances of success after 4 hours post-injury are low. A simple first-aid measure is to keep the tooth in the child's mouth if they are cooperative (saliva is protective) or in a cup of milk, pending reimplantation. As soon as possible, the tooth should be reimplanted into the socket and held in position by the child (by occluding the mouth or with a finger) or by an adult, until the on-call OFM doctor can come and fix it in position.

Avulsion of a permanent tooth is an emergency!

Wobbly or chipped teeth

Most of these injuries can be seen by the patient's own dentist, the next working day. Where there is either suspicion of alveolar fracture, or significant difficulty with occlusion, discuss with the OFM service.

CHIN LACERATIONS

Wounds under the chin occur frequently, when children fall forwards or come off a bicycle. They can nearly always be repaired with adhesive strips, even if they are gaping. Assess for mandibular fracture (see 'Fractures of the mandible').

FACIAL FRACTURES

'Blow-out' fracture of the inferior orbital margin

This injury occurs when an object, e.g. a small ball, hits the eye rather than the zygoma. It is uncommon in children. The contents of the orbit are pushed down through the orbital floor, since this is the weakest point. There may be an associated hyphaema (see 'Hyphaema', above). The inferior rectus muscle becomes trapped, causing diplopia on upward gaze.

The classical appearance on X-ray is a ball of proptosed tissue, described as a 'tear-drop' visible in the maxillary antrum (Figure 4.1). All 'blow-out' fractures must be discussed with an ophthalmologist immediately. It is crucial that the child does not blow their nose; this can severely worsen the entrapment of soft tissues.

Fractures of the zygomatic complex

Fractures of the zygoma (Figure 4.2) are also unusual in children, and usually associated with quite severe injury, or a punch. The hallmark signs of zygomatic fracture are unilateral epistaxis, swelling and bruising of the area, subconjunctival haemorrhage (the posterior border of which cannot be seen) and loss of sensation in the distribution of the infraorbital nerve (around the cheek, nose, gum and lip on the affected side). In this age group it is best to ask advice, the same day, from the OFM service.

Fractures of the mandible

History

Fractures of the mandible (Figure 4.3) are uncommon in children, and occur most often with a fall onto the point of the chin. They may be

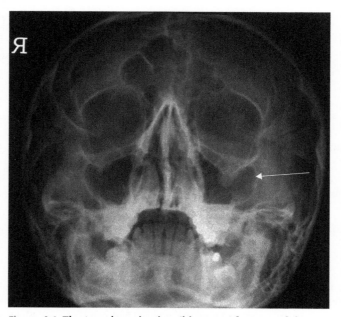

 Figure 4.1 **The tear-drop sign in a 'blow-out' fracture of the orbit.**

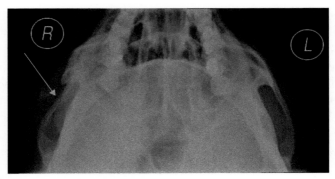

 Figure 4.2 Fractured zygoma.

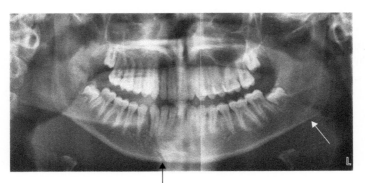

 Figure 4.3 Mandible fractured in two places.

 OPGs can be hard to interpret. Try to trace any lucent line beyond the edge of the bone to see if it relates to an overlying structure. This image shows bilateral mandibular fractures involving the roots of the right canine and the left wisdom tooth.

caused by a punch in adolescents. Remember that the mandible is a ring-type structure, so it may fracture in two places, as in Figure 4.3, even with one point of impact, e.g. fracture of the body with associated fracture of the condylar neck.

Examination

The hallmarks of mandibular fracture are pain, swelling, malocclusion of the teeth, poor mouth opening and bruising (particularly around the gum or sublingually). There may be anaesthesia in the distribution of a mental nerve.

Management

Request an AP view of the mandible and an orthopantomogram view (OPG). This is performed on specialist radiological equipment that moves from one side of the mandible to the other over 30 seconds or so. Refer all fractures to the OFM service.

CHAPTER 5

NECK AND BACK INJURIES

INTRODUCTION

Spinal injuries are rare in children, and are usually associated with high-impact injury mechanisms such as a pedestrian hit by a car. Although serious injury is rare, minor injury to the neck and back is common, and it is important to feel secure in assessing severity.

STOP Consider the mechanism of injury. Does this need a full trauma survey, not just a spine assessment?

Children may sustain fractures and/or dislocations of the spine, which may or may not be stable, or associated with cord injury. A history of transient neurological symptoms such as numbness or tingling (seconds or minutes) is not uncommon, and usually indicates minor cord contusion.

In the cervical spine, it is not uncommon for children to sustain cord injury without fracture, as a result of ligamentous injury. In fact, immediately following impact the ligaments can return to their normal position, making diagnosis very difficult. Plain films may appear normal, and the injury is only visible on CT or MRI scan. If cord injury is present, this may be called 'SCIWORA': Spinal Cord Injury Without Radiographic Abnormality.

Thoracic and lumbar fractures are also uncommon in childhood. Typical mechanisms would include falling from a height, or a vehicle crash without an appropriate seat-belt.

SPINAL IMMOBILISATION

Cervical spinal immobilisation in practice is difficult in children, and is managed differently around the world. In general, an alert child who is freely moving their arms and legs does not have an unstable injury. They may need imaging but do not need immobilisation. Immobilisation is disorientating and uncomfortable, and upsets children, making the rest of the examination difficult. If a child is very agitated, immobilisation may be harmful, as the body is pivoting on the neck. A child with torticollis following neck trauma may have a vertebral injury (such as unifacet dislocation) but will be stabilising their own neck and should not be forced to straighten their head.

A child with a significant mechanism of injury and reduced consciousness level should have manual immobilisation until their head can be protected from movement with blocks or blankets either side. Manual immobilisation can be done in either of two ways (Figures 5.1 and 5.2). A hard collar is not required, and can be difficult to adjust to the right size in children. A child in this situation who requires transport to hospital, however, should receive full immobilisation (Figure 5.3) until they are in a controlled environment (inside the hospital). A vacuum mattress (Figure 5.4), sometimes with additional padding around the head and neck, is a device in which the child lies in a neutral position, and which 'shrinks to fit' as the air is sucked out. This is an alternative to full immobilisation.

The child may arrive from the pre-hospital phase on a spinal board (Figure 5.5). This is an extrication device which is used in the pre-hospital phase. The child should be log-rolled off this hard board soon after arrival (see Chapter 15) and allowed to lie on a firm surface such as a trolley. A better alternative is a bivalve 'scoop' stretcher (Figure 5.6); this undoes at the top and the bottom and pulls out from the child's sides, thus avoiding the need for log-rolling.

Video 5.1   Log roll off spinal board: https://youtu.be/9N1C5HLttJ4

Thoracic and lumbar spinal immobilisation is achieved by lying the child on a firm, flat surface such as a hospital trolley. If a child is uncooperative with this and wants to sit up, they are highly unlikely to have a thoracic or lumbar fracture.

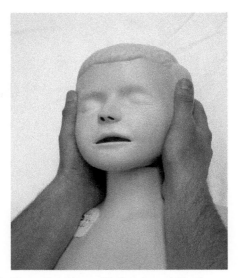

Figure 5.1 Manual in-line immobilisation of C spine from below.

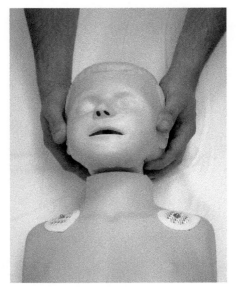

Figure 5.2 Manual in-line immobilisation of C spine from above.

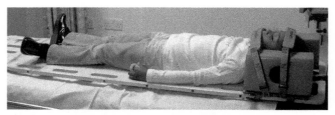

Figure 5.3 C spine immobilised on long spinal board, with blocks and straps.

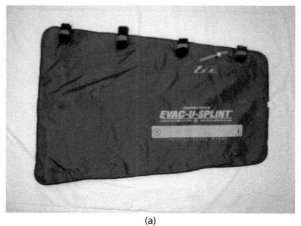

(a)

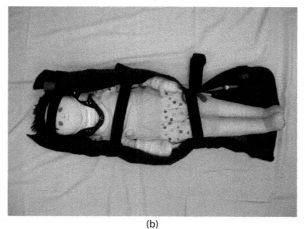

(b)

Figure 5.4 Vacuum mattress.

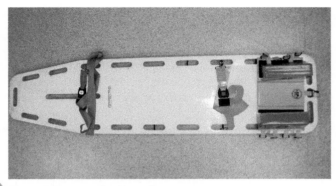

 Figure 5.5 Long spinal board.

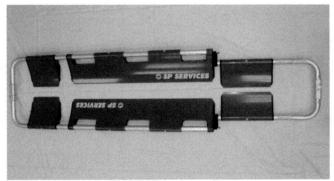

 Figure 5.6 Bivalve 'scoop' stretcher.

Clinically clearing the neck

Children hate lying flat on their backs, immobilised. Within 15 minutes of arrival, a clinician competent in clinically clearing the spine should assess the child to see if they can be allowed to mobilise; if it is not safe to do so they should be sent for imaging immediately. The rules for safe clinical clearance of the neck in children aged 10 and over are covered in several guidelines such as NEXUS, the Canadian C-Spine Rule and the UK NICE guidelines (last update 2014).

 Here is a link for the UK national guidelines on head and spinal injury (NICE): http://www.nice.org.uk/CG176

Essentially, it is important to be sure that all of the following are true:

- the child is fully conscious, orientated and able to communicate with you (drugs and/or alcohol are a contra-indication to clinical clearance)
- the mechanism of injury is not high risk (such as those listed above)
- there is no neurological deficit detectable in the arms or legs
- there is no distracting painful injury elsewhere
- there is no torticollis or abnormal posture of head
- if all the above are true, when asked, the child is able to rotate their head at least 45 degrees to the left and the right

If all the checks above are satisfactory, you are safe to remove immobilisation and let the child sit up. If your patient is reluctant to move, do not force them. Try reassurance and analgesia and reassess in half an hour. At this point, if movement is still very limited, further imaging is needed. Get senior help.

 If unable to clear the C spine clinically on the criteria above, imaging is required!

In children under 4 years, assessment will likely need to involve observation of how much the child wants to move their neck themselves, and whether they are using their arms and legs properly. In a child of this age with a minor or moderate mechanism of injury who is alert, cervical spine injury is very rare.

The only exception to this is in non-accidental injury. However, these children will tend to be under 2 years of age, and they will usually have other injuries, such as bruising, fractures or a head injury.

THE LOG-ROLL EXAMINATION OF THE THORACIC AND LUMBAR SPINE

If you suspect back injury, the principles of management are the same as the cervical spine. Consider the mechanism of injury, whether the child is alert and orientated and check for any sensory or motor deficit in the arms and legs. Generally speaking, alert children who are happy to sit up have no vertebral fracture.

In children with significant pain or a reduced consciousness level, to examine the back itself you will need to perform a controlled 'log-roll'

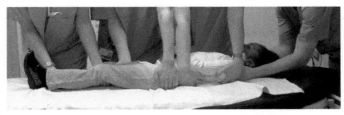

 Figure 5.7 Hand positions for a log-roll.

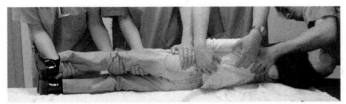

 Figure 5.8 Normal cervical spine soft tissues and alignment.

ensuring the spine remains aligned (see Figures 5.7, 5.8 and Chapter 15). Roll the child only as far as is necessary to inspect the back and palpate the whole spine firmly to localise any tenderness or pain.

Clinical examination is quite poor at detecting thoracic and lumbar fractures. If the mechanism of injury suggests that a fracture may be possible and the child can point to a midline area of their spine where they are experiencing pain, do not rely on tenderness to palpation, but consider imaging.

IMAGING

The standard X-ray views you need to request for spine injury are an anterior-posterior, a lateral and for C spine injury in children over 9 years old, an odontoid peg view. Interpretation of children's spine X-rays can be difficult even for the experienced.

Alignment is key. The lines you should follow are demonstrated in Figure 5.9a and b.

Indirect evidence of injury may be seen in cervical X-rays by assessing soft tissue swelling. The broken line in Figure 5.9b shows the diameter of normal soft tissues. Presence or absence of soft tissue swelling is an indicator of a fracture. Any deviation from normal requires radiological or senior advice, before you allow the patient to move around.

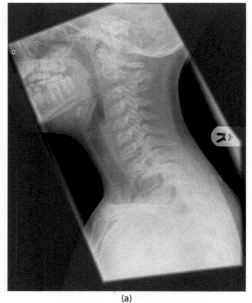

(a)

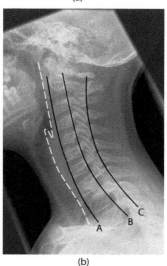

(b)

Figure 5.9 (a) Normal cervical spine (b) Normal alignment showing anterior and posterior vertebral lines (A,B) and the spinolaminar line (C). Normal soft tissue thickness (dotted line).

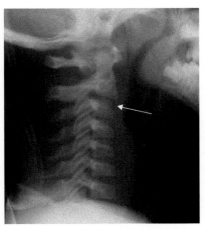

 Figure 5.10 Pseudo-subluxation of C2 on C3.

Figure 5.10 shows an example of a normal variant. In younger children there is frequently pseudo-subluxation of C2 on C3, or C3 on C4, which is emphasised in infants and young children if the film is taken horizontally with the child lying down, because of their large occiput. In addition there are multiple physeal lines and ossification centres such as the ring apophyses visible in puberty at the corners of vertebral bodies, which may be mistaken for tear-drop fractures.

If you detect a fracture, look for another, as it is possible to find multiple levels involved in spinal injuries.

CT scanning with 3D reconstruction is swift with modern scanners and is particularly useful for those ligamentous injuries which are more common in children. However, the radiation dose to the thyroid gland is significant, and senior colleagues should guide you in your decisions.

SPRAINS OF THE NECK AND BACK

Children are generally active, so injury to the neck or back is not uncommon. If a child is brought to the emergency department immobilised, go through the stages described above and if fracture is unlikely, give analgesia and review half an hour later, encouraging them to sit up. If they can do this unassisted, imaging is not necessary, unless they are in severe pain or the mechanism of injury is worrying. Treatment for soft tissue injuries involves simple painkillers, and exercises to avoid stiffness.

FRACTURES AND DISLOCATIONS OF THE SPINE

These are uncommon and largely beyond the remit of this book. Uni-facet dislocation of a cervical vertebra is a stable injury, which commonly occurs with 'a clash of heads' in sport. Dislocation of the ligaments can occur in the cervical spine, and usually involves the upper three vertebrae in young children, and the C7/T1 junction in older children.

There are two radiological phenomena worth knowing about in children: C spine dislocations are possible without any bony injury, yet can be severe enough to cause spinal cord compression. This phenomenon is known as SCIWORA, as mentioned in the Introduction. Also, the pre-vertebral soft tissue can appear relatively thick in small children. However, it should measure less than half the vertebral body at C3 and less than a full vertebral body at C6 (retrotracheal) (see Figure 5.9b). Crying, neck flexion and intubation can cause apparent soft tissue widening unrelated to spinal injury. Apparent swelling can be seen in any intubated child but in this case it is severe and related to obvious underlying fractures of C2 and C6.

There is a useful aide memoire, the '2 at 6 and 6 at 2' rule: 2 cm of soft tissue shadow anterior to C6 and 6 mm of shadow in front of C2.

NON-TRAUMATIC BACK PAIN

Be cautious in diagnosing a sprain of any part of the spine unless there is a clear and convincing history of trauma. Tumours and infections can present at any age. Acute back pain in adolescents can be the result of simple back muscle spasm and less often, acute disc prolapse, and is managed in the same way as in adults, but is uncommon.

Adolescents present with back pain symptoms more frequently than younger children. The conditions most often responsible, such as Scheuermann's disease and spondylolysis/spondylolisthesis, usually present with insidious onset or chronic symptoms. Spinal pain in children under 10 years is very unusual and should be investigated promptly. Spinal pain can also be caused by discitis (a staphylococcal infection in younger children), tuberculosis, malignancies and from repeated injury related to high levels of certain sports.

CHAPTER 6

FRACTURES AND DISLOCATIONS: GENERAL APPROACH

INTRODUCTION

Before the age of 16 around 50% of boys and 25% of girls will sustain a fracture. Dislocations, however, are uncommon in pre-pubertal children, apart from those with a collagen disorder such as Ehlers-Danlos syndrome. The bones of children differ from those of an adult in three respects (Figure 6.1):

(1) A child's bones are less brittle than those of an adult due to a higher collagen-to-bone ratio. Therefore, incomplete fractures may occur (torus or greenstick fractures).
(2) The growth plate (or physis) may bear the brunt of the injury.
(3) The periosteum in young children is very strong, and protects the bone from fracture, or can limit displacement if it does fracture (e.g. a 'toddler's' fracture of the tibia).

Buckle and torus fractures

A 'buckle' fracture describes an injury in which the cortex buckles under compression. When the buckle is circumferential it forms a compression ring or 'torus' (Latin for a doughnut shape) around the bone (Figure 6.2). It is useful to show the image to the parents and explain that although the word 'fracture' means a broken bone, it is not a break, as they would imagine.

Plastic bowing deformity

In a similar way to torus fractures, a child's bone may bend instead of breaking, but without sign of buckling of the cortex. This is called plastic deformity (Figure 6.3), and may require an experienced eye to detect on X-ray. It usually affects the radius, ulna or fibula. It will remodel back to normal over time.

Greenstick fractures

Greenstick fractures (Figure 6.4) occur because of bending forces. The cortex on the tension side breaks apart in a saw-tooth pattern whilst the

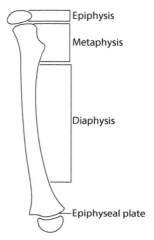

Epiphysis

Metaphysis

Diaphysis

Epiphyseal plate

Figure 6.1 Anatomy of a child's bone.

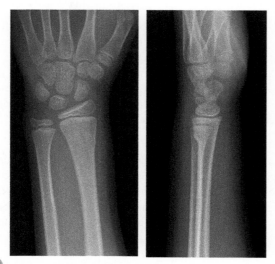

Figure 6.2 A torus fracture.

The X-ray appearances can be subtle – look for convexity in the normally concave line of the bony cortex and remember to look carefully at both views.

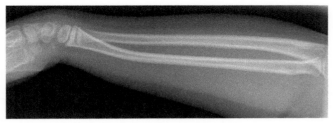

Figure 6.3 Plastic bowing deformity of the radius.

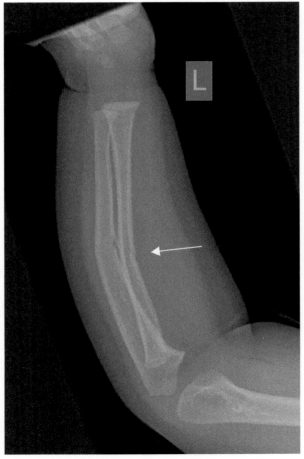

Figure 6.4 Mid-shaft greenstick fractures of the radius and ulna.

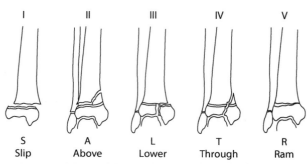

I	II	III	IV	V
S	A	L	T	R
Slip	Above	Lower	Through	Ram

 Figure 6.5 The Salter–Harris classification of physeal injuries with an aide memoire.

cortex on the opposite compression side buckles, just like a 'green stick' (young twig) when you try to break it.

Growth plate injuries

A child's bone must also have the ability to grow and achieves this by the presence of cartilaginous growth plates at the ends of long bones. The growth plate or physis (sometimes referred to as the epiphyseal plate) is a relatively weak part of the bone and is vulnerable to various patterns of fracture. These injuries were originally classified by Salter–Harris into five types (Figure 6.5). The diagram demonstrates an easy way to memorise the five types. Type II is the most common injury.

> With a clever choice of words, the Salter–Harris classification can be easily remembered, to mimic the name 'Salter.'

It is important that these injuries are identified and treated appropriately. This is especially true when the fracture breaks the continuity of the growth plate and the articular surface (types III and IV). Treatment of type III and IV fractures requires restoration of the perfect continuity of the growth plate and the articular surface (usually by internal fixation) to minimise the potential for later growth disturbance and traumatic arthritis. The type V injury is very difficult to diagnose initially, and may present as abnormal growth many months later.

Metaphyseal corner fractures

These fractures are almost pathognomonic of non-accidental injury and are difficult to spot. See Chapter 14 for full details and some examples.

GENERAL PRINCIPLES OF ASSESSMENT

History

The child's age may give a clue to the injury. For example, a fractured scaphoid bone is unusual below the age of 9; acromio-clavicular or shoulder dislocations are rare before adolescence; a toddler's fracture occurs in toddlers! When you take the history the exact mechanism of injury is important for several reasons.

Firstly, it will tell you the likelihood of a fracture and therefore help you to decide whether or not you need to ask for an X-ray. For example, falling over onto an outstretched hand is more likely to break a bone than banging against something. A direct blow can sometimes cause a fracture and/or dislocation at that site, but quite severe force would be involved. More often fractures occur as a result of indirect forces. For example, a fall on an outstretched hand may lead to a fractured distal radius, a supracondylar fracture of the elbow or a fractured clavicle.

 If significant forces are involved, e.g. child hit by car, be on your guard for any significant injury!

Secondly, the mechanism of injury will tell you whether a specific diagnosis is likely, if you know which injury patterns are associated with the various fractures. For example, a femur will only fracture with quite severe force or an awkward twist; a clavicle will break easily; a toddler's fracture is caused by a twisting mechanism. Lastly, if the story does not match up with your findings on examination or on the X-ray, then you must consider non-accidental injury.

 Is the history for this injury clear and does it match your findings? If not, consider non-accidental injury.

Examination

When examining for evidence of a fracture or dislocation, you should look, then feel, then very gently try to move the affected area, unless it is very painful.

What to look for
- Deformity (bending, rotation)
- Swelling (comparing with the opposite side helps)

- Bruising
- Any wounds
- Abnormal posture or alignment

Children can be quite deceptively calm or indeed active, despite significant injuries. Therefore limping, non-use of a limb or abnormal posture should all be taken seriously.

What to feel for

- Tenderness – it is important to try to localise this to the point of maximal tenderness, to help you with X-ray ordering and interpretation
- Deformity (comparing with the opposite side helps)
- Distal pulse/capillary refill/sensation

The more localised the tenderness, the more likely there is a fracture present. If the child is unable to localise the pain, try asking them to press around the area themselves and tell you where it hurts the most. If they are not very specific, you can then try gently pressing yourself, and offer options 'this bit or this bit?' or 'number one, number two or number three' as you try different areas. For pre-verbal children it may be difficult, but by being gentle and systematic, and sometimes repeating pressing and moving the limb whilst the child is distracted, you can usually localise the injury and avoid over-irradiating the child by ordering views of multiple bones.

How to assess movement

Give the child an opportunity to use the limb, e.g. introduce them to some toys or just ask them to copy you, and watch how the limb is held or used. Think through your joint movements so you test the full range – for example elbows can supinate and pronate, as well as flex and extend. Attempt movements of the relevant joints if pain allows.

Do not cause unnecessary pain, but at the same time you must persist to an extent. Try getting the child to show you rather than you moving the limb, and tell them that if they can just demonstrate a movement once, that's enough for you to know they can do it – for example, full elbow or knee extension. Ensure you isolate the joint movement which you are trying to test, to limit pain and to limit compensation from another joint – for example, support the wrist if you move the elbow, and vice versa.

 By being patient, trying to localise tenderness, repeating movements and using distraction, you can avoid over- ordering of X-rays or missing injuries!

X-RAYS

When to X-ray

If in doubt, have a low threshold for requesting X-rays. Young children in particular can have quite subtle signs for fractures such as greenstick fractures. Most parents will be expecting you to X-ray their child, but you have to use your experience, and explain the potential future consequences of irradiation if you consider the X-ray to be unnecessary. Use the information such as mechanism of injury and likelihood of a positive X-ray to help you.

It is better to get senior advice than over-request X-rays!

Which X-rays to request

It is crucial to order the right X-ray view if you are not to miss fractures. If in doubt, ask a radiographer for their advice, explaining the context. To ensure adequate X-rays are taken always give as much information as possible on the request card. The area you specify on your request should be as focussed as possible (see Table 6.1 to guide you). To diagnose and fully assess the injury, two films should be taken at right angles to each other; this is most usually anteroposterior and lateral views, but usually the radiographer will decide this for you. For mid-shaft, long-bone fractures, the joint above and the joint below should be seen.

Interpretation of paediatric X-rays

Interpreting paediatric X-rays comes with practice. Fractures may be very subtle and the presence of various ossification centres around joints can add to the confusion. If in doubt about an X-ray, always seek a second opinion.

In practice, most services should have a safety net system whereby a radiologist will report the film in the next couple of days and the patient can be contacted if something has been missed. If you explain this to the parents at the time, they will tend to leave your consultation more reassured, and if they are called back they will appreciate the call and understand the context.

There is a useful website to help you decide if an X-Ray is normal for a child of a certain age, or abnormal. See https://radiopaedia.org.

Table 6.1 **Requests for radiographic studies**

Body area	Appropriate request	Injury or fracture (#) suspected
Upper limb	Shoulder	Ruptured acromio-clavicular joint or dislocation head of humerus
	Clavicle	# clavicle
	Humerus	# shaft humerus
	Elbow	# supracondylar, # of either epicondyle, # radial head or neck, # olecranon
	Forearm	# shaft radius/ulna
	Wrist	# distal radius/ulna
	Scaphoid views	# or dislocation of any carpal bones
	Hand	# metacarpals
	Finger	Finger down to and including MCPJ
Lower limb	Pelvis	Any hip pathology. If you are looking for SUFE add 'frog leg lateral' to your request
	Femur	# femur
	Knee	Dislocated or # patella, # of knee itself
	Tibia and fibula	# tibia or fibula
	Ankle	# medial or lateral malleolus, or distal tibia
	Foot	All bones of foot, except calcaneum
	Calcaneum	Calcaneum
Spine	Peg view	Odontoid peg and C1
	Lateral C spine	C1–T1
	Anteroposterior C spine	C1–T1
	Thoracic spine	T1–T12
	Lumbar spine	L1–L5

GENERAL PRINCIPLES OF MANAGEMENT

General principles

Fractures and dislocations are painful so ensure the child has adequate analgesia as soon as they reach you (see Chapter 2). You should immobilise the injury from the outset, whether with a splint, plaster cast or sling, because this will help a great deal with pain. Pain management is also very important for discharge.

Most injuries will require immobilisation to prevent pain and promote healing. Simple fractures, which have no axial rotation and only minor degrees of angulation and displacement, will simply require a plaster cast and orthopaedic clinic follow-up. Immobilisation may be either by bandage, splint or a plaster cast, depending on the location and degree of displacement.

Some fractures and dislocations will require either manipulation under deep sedation or general anaesthesia (manipulation under anaesthesia, shortened to MUA), some structural support from pins or screws such as K wires or an open reduction with internal fixation (ORIF). These may include fractures with:

- Significant clinical deformity
- Axial rotation
- Significant angulation (usually > 20°, but the upper limit is age dependent)
- Significant displacement
- Growth plate fractures
- Irreducible dislocations
- Fracture dislocations

There may be other reasons for immediate referral and hospital admission. One of these is simply for pain control. Another reason is if there is a risk of, or evidence of:

- Compartment syndrome (see Chapter 3)
- Neurological or vascular compromise
- Severe swelling needing elevation (e.g. hand injuries)

Dislocations

Dislocated joints are very painful, but the pain is greatly decreased as soon as the joint is reduced, so these patients must be prioritised for reduction of the joint, which may require procedural sedation or opiate analgesia (see Chapter 2) when large joints are involved. Dislocations of fingers and the patella usually only require simpler strategies.

Dislocations are more likely to cause neurovascular damage and joint reduction might possibly cause damage, so carefully document your neurovascular examination both before and afterwards!

Open fractures

Open (also known as compound) fractures need to be thoroughly cleaned under operating theatre conditions as soon as possible after injury. If you suspect an open fracture, dress the wound with an antiseptic-soaked dressing, and give parenteral anti-staphylococcal antibiotics. Prevent other people from continually disturbing the wound – a digital camera image can be invaluable in this situation.

Suspect an open fracture if there is any kind of wound overlying, or near to, the fracture. Refer to orthopaedics immediately!

There are evidence-based national recommendations for the management of open fractures of the lower limb in the UK. These can be freely accessed through BOAST (British Orthopaedic Association Standards for Trauma) document 4: https://www.boa.ac.uk/wp-content/uploads/2014/12/BOAST-4.pdf.

PLASTER CASTS

In the first 24 hours after injury the area is likely to swell, so a full plaster is not usually applied. The plaster should surround about 75% of the limb, allowing a gap for swelling to occur. This is called a 'backslab'. Plasters can be made out of plaster of Paris (POP). This is cheap and fairly easy to learn how to apply. Synthetic polymer materials are lighter in weight, and can be purchased in attractive colours! Because they are more expensive and are more difficult to make into a backslab, most departments apply a POP backslab initially, then offer an appointment a day or two later for conversion to a full plaster.

If a plaster cast has been applied, ensure that the family knows it should not get wet. They must also understand to return if the plaster is uncomfortable or painful, if the limb becomes swollen, if there is coldness, tingling or numbness distally or if the cast is rubbing the skin. If these symptoms occur, the plaster should be removed in order to inspect the underlying limb. That is, unless there has been a MUA or ORIF, in which case orthopaedic advice should be obtained before moving the plaster.

CHAPTER 7

INJURIES OF THE SHOULDER TO WRIST

INTRODUCTION

For general principles of assessment, investigation and management of fractures and dislocations in children, see Chapter 6. Hand injuries are covered in Chapter 8. Fractures of the upper limb are much more common than the lower limb.

The most common fractures are of the distal radius and clavicle. The commonest mechanism of injury in all age groups is a 'fall onto the outstretched hand' (FOOSH), in other words the protective reflex that we all have, to break a fall. In children the exact mechanism of injury is often less clear than when taking a history from an adult.

THE SHOULDER

Clavicle fracture

Assessment

Fracture of the clavicle usually occurs following a fall. It is common throughout childhood. Birth injuries can occur, and may not present for a few weeks – often when a lump (callus) appears. Toddlers may not be brought to medical attention for a day or two after injury, as they tend to only have mild symptoms. While delay in presentation should normally ring 'alarm bells' (see Chapter 14), it is quite common with clavicular fractures. In young children focal tenderness may not be clear, and reasonable arm function may be preserved, however abduction of the arm is usually painful. If the child can abduct beyond 90° fracture is unlikely and X-rays are not needed. Occasionally, tenting of the skin over a displaced fracture occurs. This looks dramatic but does not need same-day referral.

X-ray

Most fractures are fairly obvious. The middle portion of the clavicle is most commonly broken. Distal clavicular fractures are covered in acromio-clavicular injury (Figure 7.1). Young children may have a greenstick fracture (Figure 7.2), which may be difficult to see because the clavicle curves naturally.

Management

Apply a broad-arm sling (see Chapter 15), and arrange orthopaedic clinic follow-up. If a toddler will not keep a sling on do not worry, simply

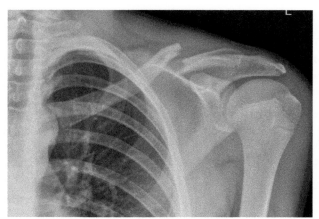

 Figure 7.1 Displaced fracture of the clavicle.

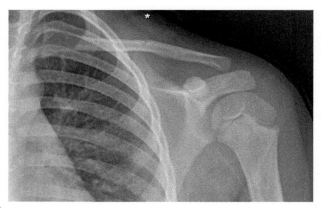

 Figure 7.2 Greenstick fracture of the clavicle.

reassure the parents that the bone will heal well. Advise all parents that a lump may be present after healing, which will reduce in size over 6–12 months.

Shoulder dislocation

Gleno-humeral dislocation is uncommon in children, and in pre-teenage years tends only to occur with severe force, during fits, or in those with connective tissue disorders. Younger teenagers have a high risk of recurrent dislocation, often with no trauma – simply on reaching or stretching.

Assessment

The deformity is usually obvious, and pain is severe. There is a palpable gap below the acromion. There is no need to move the arm to test range of movement. There may be associated sensory loss over the deltoid area due to compression of the axillary nerve, which usually resolves once the joint is relocated.

A small subset of patients present with repeated dislocation, often with little or no trauma, because of a combination of ligament laxity and dysfunctional muscle control around the shoulder joint. Such patients should be referred for orthopaedic review.

X-ray

There are two types of dislocation – anterior (more than 90% in children) and the much less common posterior dislocation (more likely during a seizure, during the strong muscle spasm). In Figure 7.3 you can see that the humeral head is displaced inferior and anterior to the glenoid. Associated fractures are unusual in children.

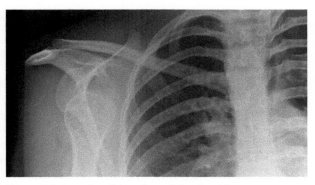

 Figure 7.3 Anterior dislocation of the shoulder.

In a posterior dislocation the humeral head can appear to be in joint on the AP view, as it may move directly posteriorly. One clue is the 'light-bulb' appearance, when the normal slightly asymmetrical appearance of the humeral head (like the head of a walking stick) becomes more symmetrical, like a light bulb, due to internal rotation. A widened joint space is another sign, with no overlap of the humeral head on the glenoid. In many cases a second view is needed to make the diagnosis. Figure 7.4 shows a posterior dislocation in a child who had recurrent shoulder dislocations.

Posterior dislocations are very easily missed on the standard AP shoulder view as the humeral head often moves directly posteriorly. Note the subtle light bulb sign on the AP view and the obvious posterior displacement on the axial view.

Management

Analgesia is the priority (see Chapter 2). However, the best analgesia is reduction of the dislocation. The sooner this is done, the easier the procedure. An X-ray should be performed first, though, to see if it is an anterior (>90%) or posterior dislocation, and whether there is an associated fracture (in which case orthopaedic referral is recommended).

Reduction of the dislocation depends on adequate muscle relaxation. Much of this can be achieved through psychological measures (Chapter 2) so sedation is not always necessary. Relatively painless joint reduction can be achieved with nitrous oxide (Entonox®), an intra-articular injection of lignocaine (see Chapter 15) and the slow external rotation method. Ideally the intra-articular block should be performed as soon as possible after the patient arrives, and before X-ray. Self-reduction is possible after analgesia, sometimes during movements such as positioning for an X-ray, or if lying prone with the arm dangling down; this can work for recurrent dislocations. There is no place for brute force.

Slow external rotation is the gentlest method of reduction. Stand, or preferably sit, next to the child with them sitting up and relaxing back. Take their elbow and support it gently on one hand and use your other hand to hold the child's hand. Spend plenty of time gaining the child's trust and getting them to relax their shoulder muscles. Very slowly start external rotation. Over 5–10 minutes you are aiming for 90° of external rotation. At around this point the shoulder will slip back into the joint, usually with a palpable clunk. There are many other methods of reduction so if this does not work, seek senior advice.

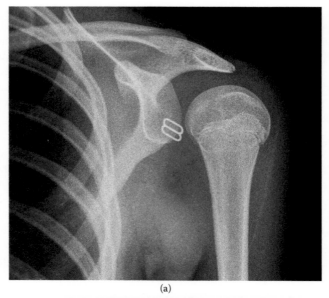

(a)

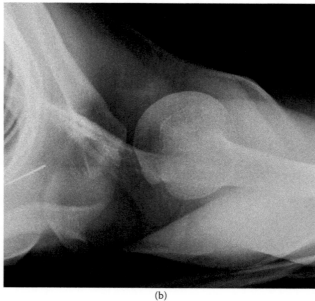

(b)

Figure 7.4 Posterior dislocation of the shoulder
(a) AP and (b) axial views.

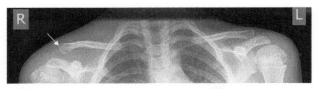

 Figure 7.5 Acromio-clavicular joint disruption.

After reduction, place the arm in a broad arm sling (see Chapter 15), and X-ray again to check the shoulder is fully reduced. Arrange for orthopaedic follow-up within a week or two.

Acromio-clavicular joint injury

Assessment
This injury (Figure 7.5) usually occurs in teenagers, following a fall directly onto the shoulder. After puberty there is true rupture of the ligaments but before that age, the apparent A-C dislocation is caused by a fracture through the epiphysis. Tenderness ± swelling is usually localised to the point where the acromion meets the clavicle. Deformity may be seen and can initially be confused with gleno-humeral dislocation.

X-rays
These are necessary only if deformity is seen.

Management
Symptomatic management in a broad arm sling (see Chapter 15) for a week or two is usually sufficient. Arrange follow-up in an orthopaedic clinic for those who have visible deformity.

THE UPPER ARM

Proximal humerus fracture

Assessment
Fracture of the neck of the humerus occurs by falling onto the shoulder itself, or onto the outstretched hand. It is not a very common fracture in children. However it is not an uncommon area to get a bone cyst so sometimes a pathological fracture may occur with quite minor trauma. Ability to abduct the arm beyond 90° makes a fracture unlikely.

X-ray
X-ray findings may be subtle. Look for growth plate fractures or a buckle/greenstick fracture (Figure 7.6).

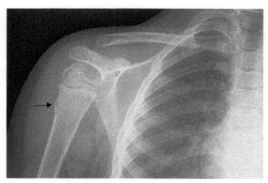

 Figure 7.6 Buckle fracture of proximal humerus.

Management

Refer displaced growth plate fractures, pathological fractures or angulation greater than 20° for an immediate orthopaedic opinion. Otherwise, apply a collar and cuff (see Chapter 15) and arrange clinic follow-up.

Humeral shaft fracture

Assessment

Fracture of the humeral shaft is uncommon. Clinical diagnosis is usually straightforward. Spiral fractures in infants are the exception to this. They may present with just reluctance to use the arm. This type of fracture is highly suspicious of child abuse. See Figure 7.7 as an example.

X-ray

X-ray may reveal a buckle fracture, transverse fracture, spiral fracture or pathological fracture. The proximal humerus is the most common site for a simple bone cyst and these often present after a pathological fracture.

> STOP   A spiral fracture of the humerus is highly likely to indicate non-accidental injury (see Chapter 14)!

Management

For fractures with neurological deficit or displacement, refer for an immediate orthopaedic opinion. Place the remainder (non-spiral fractures) in a collar and cuff (see Chapter 15) and arrange orthopaedic clinic follow-up.

>   Refer spiral fractures immediately to orthopaedics and consider child protection issues!

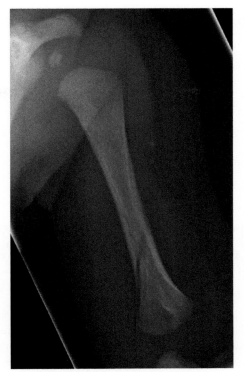

 Figure 7.7 Spiral fracture of the humerus due to non-accidental injury.

THE ELBOW

Normal or abnormal?

The many different ossification centres appearing at different ages around the elbow make interpretation of children's X-rays particularly difficult. It is helpful to have a working knowledge of these ossification centres. The acronym 'CRITOE' is often used to remember the order the centres appear (see Table 7.1). Figure 7.8 shows where these are in the elbow. If in doubt, check a radiology textbook, or consult a senior.

 There is a useful website to help you decide if an X-Ray is normal for a child of a certain age, or abnormal. See https://radiopaedia.org.

Table 7.1 The 'CRITOE' acronym for order of appearance of elbow ossification centres.

Ossification Centre	Age
C: Capitellum	1
R: Radial head	3
I: Internal (medial) epicondyle	5
T: Trochlea	7
O: Olecranon	9
E: External (lateral) epicondyle	11

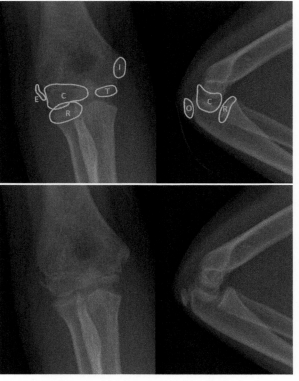

Figure 7.8 Elbow ossification centres highlighted.

As a broad rule of thumb, centres appear about every two years. Knowing the order in which they appear helps you decide whether a small fragment is an immature ossification centre or an avulsion fracture. Avulsion fractures in the elbow can be very important, in orthopaedic terms.

Another clue to help you detect a fracture is the presence of a joint effusion, which makes a fracture much more likely. On examination swelling may be seen, but this can be quite subtle. The best way to pick up swelling clinically is to position both the child's arms symmetrically (ideally at 90°) and compare the dimples on each side.

On X-ray an effusion is detected by a positive 'fat pad sign' on the lateral view. On a normal lateral elbow view a small dark area of fat is present just anterior to the humerus (Figure 7.9). This overlies the joint capsule, and flexing the elbow makes it visible. When there is a joint effusion the anterior fat pad becomes elevated away from the humerus, and the posterior fat pad which is normally hidden (stretched flat when the arm is bent 90°) is revealed (Figure 7.10). The fat pad sign is suggestive of an intra-articular fracture. However, the absence of a fat pad does not rule out a fracture. Use your clinical examination to guide your management.

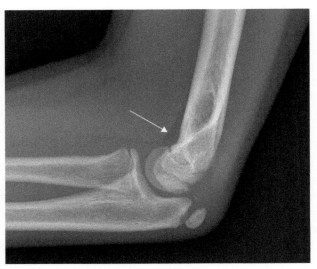

Figure 7.9 Normal anterior fat pad seen as a small lucency.

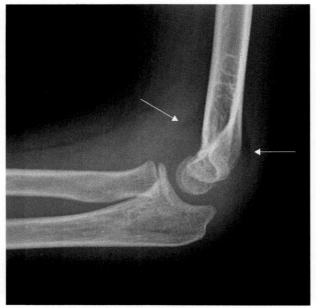

 Figure 7.10 Abnormal fat pads implying joint effusion.

Supracondylar humeral fracture

Assessment

This a common fracture in children, with a peak age at about 7 years old. It represents about 80% of elbow fractures. It is generally caused by a fall. There is usually swelling (see previous section on detection) which may be mild, or severe with deformity. It is extremely important to examine and record the distal neurological and vascular status of the arm. This fracture is associated with vascular and neurological injury and can lead to compartment syndrome (see Chapter 3).

The fracture can impinge on the brachial artery, the anterior interosseous branch of the median nerve and the radial or the ulnar nerve. Examine the radial pulse volume and the capillary refill and compare with the opposite side. Ask the child if they have pins and needles, or any numbness anywhere. It is important to assess sensory and motor function before any treatment is given. This can be difficult in injured children, especially where motor function is concerned. It is sometimes helpful to ask the child to copy you giving a 'thumbs up' sign (radial nerve motor supply), a 'starfish' spread of the fingers (ulna nerve motor supply) and an 'OK' sign with the thumb and index finger (median nerve, anterior interosseous branch, motor supply). Further information on neurological assessment can be found in Chapter 8. If you find any abnormality, motor or sensory, refer immediately to orthopaedics.

Check circulation and neurological function!

Moving the elbow can cause ischaemia!

X-ray

There is a range of possible X-ray findings. There may be a simple greenstick fracture, which may be difficult to detect, although a joint effusion is usually present. At the opposite extreme, there may be significant displacement of the distal fragment posteriorly (Figure 7.11). In displaced fractures, the distal fragment is displaced posteriorly over 90% of the time, and anteriorly in fewer than 10% of fractures.

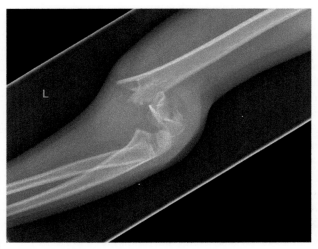

 Figure 7.11 A displaced supracondylar fracture.

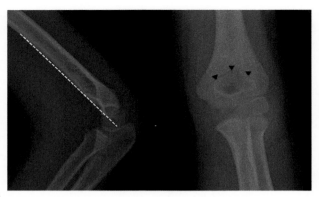

 Figure 7.12 A subtle supracondylar fracture.

 The anterior humeral line does intersect the capitellum, but slightly anterior to its middle third; this alerts you to the fracture and we can see the fracture on the AP view.

To detect subtle fractures (Figure 7.12) it is worth knowing about the anterior humeral line. This is a line drawn along the anterior surface of the distal humerus on a true lateral view. Normally this intersects the middle third of the capitellum. If the distal humerus is displaced backwards, it will intersect more anteriorly, or not at all.

Management

If there are signs of ischaemia, after appropriate analgesia (see Chapter 2) it may be necessary to move the elbow and partly reduce the fracture by gentle traction and extension, to restore some circulation. This is best done by an orthopaedic surgeon. Displaced fractures are likely to need surgery. In the absence of displacement or neurovascular signs the child is treated with an above-elbow plaster backslab. Refer to the orthopaedic clinic for follow-up.

Dislocation of the elbow

Assessment

Dislocation of the elbow is uncommon in children and usually affects those over 11 years. On examination the deformity is obvious, with substantial swelling and severe pain. Assess for neurovascular deficit in the same way as supracondylar fractures.

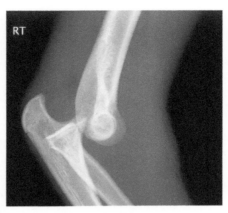

 Figure 7.13 **Elbow dislocation.**

X-ray
This will typically show a postero-lateral dislocation (Figure 7.13). Associated fractures may occur, typically the medial epicondyle.

Management
The elbow joint will require reduction as soon as possible, usually under general anaesthesia. If the circulation is affected get senior help immediately.

Medial epicondyle injury

Assessment
This fracture constitutes around 10% of elbow fractures and is often associated with a dislocated elbow (see the previous section). There are a variety of mechanisms of injury. On examination, there will be tenderness over the prominence of the medial (ulnar side) epicondyle and likely swelling (see the section 'Normal or abnormal?'). In particular, assess ulnar nerve function.

X-ray
There may be minimal or moderate displacement of the medial epicondylar apophysis (Figure 7.14). In severe injury, the medial epicondyle may become trapped in the elbow joint. It is easy to mistake the medial epicondyle within the joint for the capitellum.

Management
Refer to orthopaedics if the medial epiphysis is displaced or there is evidence of ulnar nerve damage. For undisplaced fractures, place in a collar and cuff (see Chapter 15) and arrange orthopaedic clinic follow-up.

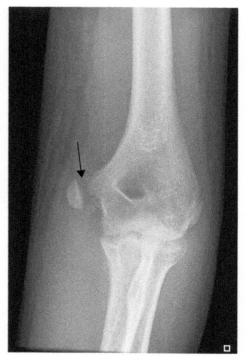

 Figure 7.14 A medial epicondylar fracture.

If the child is over 6 years old and the medial epicondylar ossification centre cannot be seen on the AP view (see the section on CRITOE), assume that it has been displaced and lies within the joint.

Lateral condyle injury

Assessment

This constitutes around 15% of elbow fractures, and is caused by a fall. On examination there will be tenderness on the prominence of the lateral (radial side) condyle. Unlike the other elbow injuries we have discussed, this is not usually associated with neurovascular problems, but it can be associated with growth problems. These fractures often break the continuity of the surface of the distal humerus and commonly require internal fixation.

X-ray

Although the fracture often includes a large chunk of unossified cartilage, X-rays may appear innocent with just a sliver of bone broken from the

 Look for subtle slivers or pieces of bone – they are significant.

lateral humeral metaphysis just above the capitellum ossification centre (Figure 7.15).

Management

Displaced fractures should be referred immediately to orthopaedics. Undisplaced fractures can be placed in an above-elbow backslab and referred to an orthopaedic clinic.

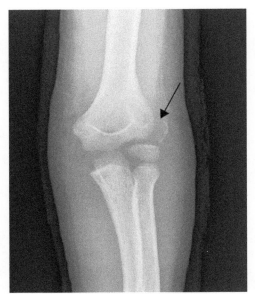

 Figure 7.15 A lateral condyle fracture.

Olecranon fracture

Assessment

These rare fractures are usually due to direct trauma, and are typically seen in teenagers. Following a direct blow to the elbow children are often tender over this area since there is little cushioning but there is no fracture. If the olecranon is truly fractured, a large amount of generalised elbow swelling is present (Figure 7.16).

X-ray

It is easy to confuse the normal epiphysis with a fracture. The normal olecranon apophysis appears between the ages of 8 and 11 and fuses by the age of 14. Seek senior advice if unsure.

 Most of the time you are just seeing a normal growth plate!

Management

A truly fractured olecranon fracture may well need internal fixation, so get immediate orthopaedic advice.

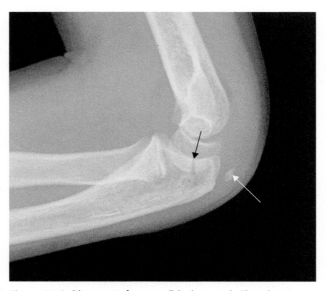

 Figure 7.16 Olecranon fracture (black arrow). The olecranon apophysis is normal (white arrow).

Radial head/neck fractures

Assessment

Radial neck fractures are relatively common in children, and are caused by a fall. Radial head fractures are more common in adults. Most fractures in children are of a Salter–Harris II type. Greenstick fractures may also occur.

Pain is often vague in distribution and referred to the whole forearm. Localising the injury can be tricky, but the clues are pain on supination and pronation of the forearm, difficulty in fully extending the elbow and tenderness at a point between the lateral epicondyle and the point of the olecranon, 1 cm distally. You can feel the radial head at this point – it moves during pronation and supination. There may or may not be mild swelling (this may be subtle, see the section 'Normal or abnormal?').

X-ray

These fractures may be difficult to detect on X-ray. The presence of a joint effusion, as indicated by a positive fat pad sign (see the section 'Normal or abnormal?') should give you a clue. Similarly, once you are thinking of it, you will notice the abnormality of the radial neck when you take care to look at the image carefully. Radial head fractures can occur in teenagers. Figures 7.17 and 7.18 are fairly classical.

Management

Place in a collar and cuff (see Chapter 15) and arrange orthopaedic clinic follow-up. Although relatively rare, displaced or significantly angulated radial neck/head fractures need immediate referral and sometimes require realignment and or fixation.

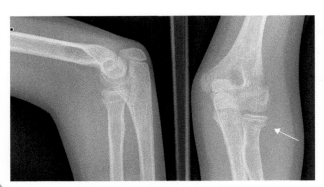

Figure 7.17 Radial neck greenstick fracture.

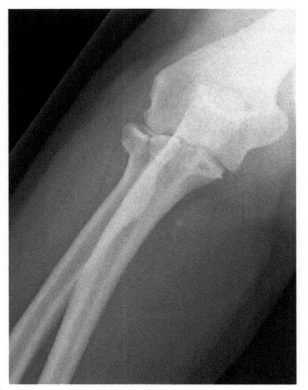

Figure 7.18 Radial head fracture.

The 'pulled' elbow

Assessment

A 'pulled' elbow is a common injury and occurs mainly in the 1–3-year age group (range 6 months to 4 years). It is caused by a sudden longitudinal pull on the arm. This mechanism of injury causes a small tear in the distal insertion of the annular ligament, and the periosteum and the head of the radius becomes entrapped in the joint. Some children are especially prone to this, so there may be previous episodes of the same injury. The ligament tightens as the child gets older so the problem is uncommon after 3 years old.

The typical situation that leads to a pulled elbow occurs when the child's hand is being held as the child is either pulled during play or away from danger, or if the child themselves pulls away. As the injury is usually 'inflicted' by a third party, the history may not be forthcoming due to feelings of guilt, or may be ascribed to a fall initially. While a changing history should normally make you very concerned about abusive injury (see Chapter 14), in this situation it is driven by guilt and in fact this injury can occur very easily, without excessive force being applied. Reassurance should be given to those present, since feelings are often running high!

The arm usually lies limp and partially flexed by the child's side. The child will use the other arm, and often appears to be playing happily. On examination, tenderness to palpation is often not elicited. Check the clavicle and the distal radius (without moving the elbow) to exclude these other common injuries. If slight elbow movement causes pain then a pulled elbow is the likely diagnosis in this age group. If both the history and the age group are completely classical, no X-ray is required, and you can go ahead and manipulate the elbow. However, if there is any uncertainty, X-ray first to exclude a fracture.

Management

Manipulating the elbow (see Chapter 15) is a simple procedure which usually gives satisfyingly rapid resolution of symptoms. You will upset the child so leave them alone with their parent and some toys and review the child after 10 minutes. Most will be using the arm happily and can go home.

If the child is still not using the arm (which is more common in older toddlers and repeat dislocators) you can have one more attempt, but if this does not seem to work it may be because the child is still sore, or has memory of the pain and is avoiding using the arm, or it is not yet reduced. Advise the parents that spontaneous reduction will usually take place and place the arm in a broad arm sling (see Chapter 15). If they are still not using the arm in 48 hours' time they should return for review.

Advise the parents in the future to avoid games that involve pulling (e.g. swinging between two adults). A pull may however be unavoidable, for example if the child starts to run across a road. Some children present with repeated dislocations as it is not always possible to avoid a pull injury. Parents of repeat dislocators may be happy to be taught the reduction technique. This kind of 'recurrent injury' is not a child protection issue. You may have to explain the condition to colleagues such as social workers.

Mid-shaft fractures of the radius and/or ulna

During a fall, both the radius and ulna can sustain mid-shaft fractures, but this is quite an unusual injury. With direct trauma, for example landing on a sharp edge or struck in self-defence, it is possible to fracture the mid-shaft of the ulna in isolation. However, this injury is relatively uncommon. Beware fracture dislocations of the forearm (see the next section).

Assessment

Fractures of the forearm bones are commonly associated with significant angulation and displacement (Figure 7.19).

Management

For greenstick fractures, up to 30° of angulation can remodel in a toddler. In teenagers, no more than 10° is acceptable. If the angulation is acceptable, place the arm in an above-elbow backslab and refer to an orthopaedic clinic within a day or two. Refer all other fractures for immediate orthopaedic advice.

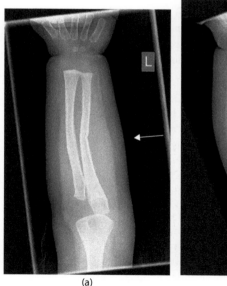 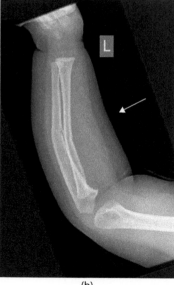

(a)   (b)

Figure 7.19 (a) AP of mid-shaft greenstick fractures of the radius and ulna, (b) lateral view of mid-shaft greenstick fractures of the radius and ulna.

Fracture dislocations of the forearm

The radius and ulna form a loop. Therefore if one breaks and the other does not, the other has probably dislocated. There are two patterns of fracture dislocation: the Monteggia and the Galeazzi.

Monteggia injury

In a Monteggia injury, there is a fracture of the ulna, with an associated dislocation of the radial head (Figure 7.20). In a normal child a longitudinal line drawn through the radius and out through the radial head (the radio-capitellar line) should point to the capitellum in all views of the elbow. If it does not, there is a radial head dislocation. Monteggia fractures with radial head subluxation are commonly overlooked.

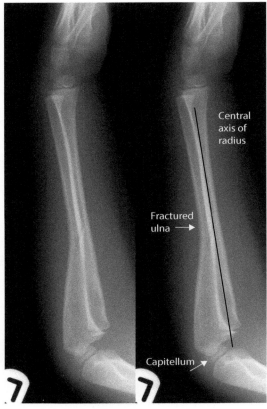

Figure 7.20 A Monteggia injury.

Always check the radio-capitellar line if you see an ulnar fracture. Here you can see that it is abnormal.

Galeazzi injury

Galeazzi injuries (Figure 7.21) occur in teenagers and are rare. There is a fracture of the shaft of radius, associated with a dislocation of the distal ulna.

Management

Refer all fracture dislocations of the radius and ulna for an immediate orthopaedic opinion.

THE WRIST

Distal radius fracture

Assessment

Fracture of the distal radius is one of the commonest injuries in all age groups, usually occurring after a fall on the outstretched hand. Signs may be subtle, for example in a torus fracture there may be only slight local tenderness, particularly in a young child, and a fairly good range of movement. Essentially, if any child points to the distal radius when asked where it hurts, an X-ray will be worthwhile in the majority of cases!

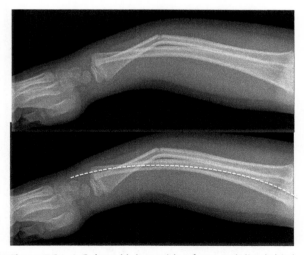

Figure 7.21 A Galeazzi injury with a fractured distal third of the radius and a dislocation of the distal ulna.

Note the plastic bowing of the ulna in this image.

If you see a shaft of radius fracture, always look to see if the gap between the distal ulna and the carpal bones looks normal.

X-ray

Findings on X-ray vary from a simple undisplaced greenstick or torus fracture, or growth plate fracture (see Chapter 6), to severe angulated, displaced fractures of both distal radius and ulna. See Figures 7.22 through 7.24.

Management

Refer immediately to orthopaedics if the fracture is angulated or displaced. Up to 25° of angulation can remodel in a toddler. In teenagers, more than 10° is unacceptable. For simple, undisplaced fractures, place in a forearm plaster of Paris backslab, or just a rigid removable splint (the ones with

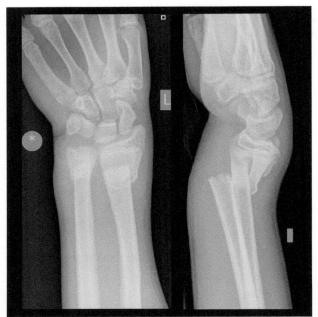

 Figure 7.22 Displaced fracture of distal radius and ulna.

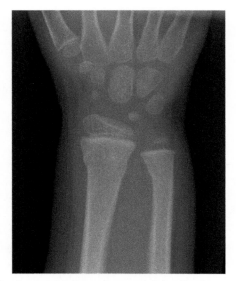

Figure 7.23 Torus fracture of the distal radius and ulna.

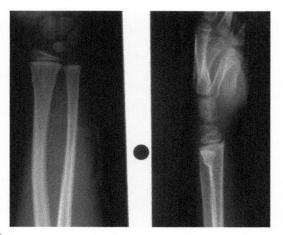

Figure 7.24 Subtle torus fracture of the distal radius.

The torus fracture is barely seen here on the AP view, as just a slight convexity of the distal radius. However, if you look carefully at the lateral view you see a much more obvious step in the cortex.

sticky straps), and arrange orthopaedic clinic follow-up. You can discharge children with undisplaced torus fractures if your orthopaedic service agrees that they require no follow-up.

Video 7.1 Application of wrist splint: https://youtu.be/vvs6W7rsYJk

Scaphoid fracture

Scaphoid fractures can only occur once the scaphoid bone has calcified, at around 9 years old. While uncommon, a missed scaphoid fracture may result in very significant disability of the wrist in future years due to non-union or avascular necrosis.

Assessment

Scaphoid injuries (Figure 7.25) are usually caused by a fall on the outstretched hand. There is usually mild swelling on the radial side of the wrist if you look carefully. The signs you should specifically examine for are:

- Tenderness in the 'anatomical snuff-box' (Figure 7.25) to gentle pressure (firm pressure will always elicit tenderness in the normal wrist as the superficial branch of the radial nerve traverses this area)

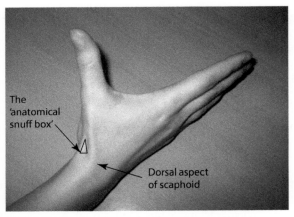

The 'anatomical snuff box'

Dorsal aspect of scaphoid

Figure 7.25 **The surface anatomy of the scaphoid.**

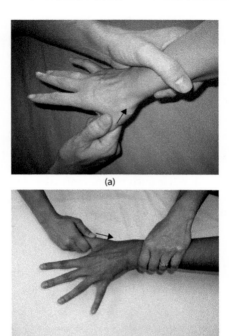

Figure 7.26 'Telescoping' the thumb to elicit pain: (a) distraction, (b) compression.

- Tenderness over the dorsal aspect of the scaphoid (Figure 7.25)
- Tenderness over the palmar aspect of the scaphoid (Figure 7.25)
- Pain at the wrist when compressing the thumb longitudinally (Figure 7.26)
- Pain during passive radial and ulnar deviation of the wrist (Figure 7.27)

Video 7.2 Scaphoid examination: https://youtu.be/PVOUSy_AS-s

X-rays

Ensure you request 'scaphoid views' (see Table 7.1). Four views are usually provided: anteroposterior, lateral and left and right obliques. In about 10% of cases the scaphoid fracture (Figure 7.28) may not be visible on initial films, and review at 10–14 days with a view to further imaging is needed if you think there is a scaphoid fracture clinically.

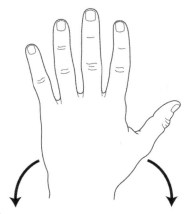

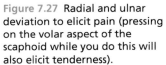

Figure 7.27 Radial and ulnar deviation to elicit pain (pressing on the volar aspect of the scaphoid while you do this will also elicit tenderness).

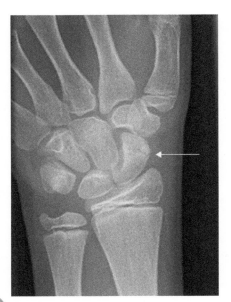

Figure 7.28 Scaphoid fracture.

Management

If you suspect a scaphoid fracture, you must treat the child as if they have one, even if no fracture has been seen on initial images. Place the wrist in a scaphoid plaster cast or a rigid splint with a thumb extension. Arrange orthopaedic clinic follow-up at 10–14 days.

THE HAND

INTRODUCTION

Hand injuries are common. Young children sustain crush injuries and burns while exploring their environment, and older children are prone to sports injuries. Most injuries are minor but the complexity and density of important structures in the hand make it vulnerable to serious, permanent injury. If a significant injury is missed, there may be enormous long-term consequences in terms of loss of function, for their hobbies or occupation. Luckily, long-term problems due to stiffness are very unlikely since young children will continue to use their hands despite injury. This is different in adults.

If in doubt about the extent of a hand injury, always seek expert advice!

Hand injuries frequently swell. Swelling causes pain and stiffness. This may be prevented by elevation to shoulder level in a 'high arm sling' (see Chapter 15), if the child will cooperate. This helps to alleviate pain, and is necessary for a day or two if swelling is present or predictable. Consult your local policy for referral procedures, since hand specialists may be part of the orthopaedic or plastic surgery services, and referral may depend on the exact nature of the injury.

Rings should always be removed on arrival to prevent swelling and ischaemia of a digit!

CLINICAL EXAMINATION

A methodical, slick system for examining hands is essential, albeit with modifications for young children. The hand is one area where you really do need to understand the underlying anatomy. Sometimes exploration under general anaesthetic is needed if a wound is deep, to check for injury to tendons or nerves. Also, important fractures can have only subtle clinical signs on examination, so have a low threshold for X-ray – the radiation dose for these views is extremely low.

Have a low threshold for X-rays! Clinical examination is not that reliable for determining the probability of a fracture!

The infant or pre-school child

Small children are unable to obey the simple commands needed to test hand function. You are therefore dependent on observation of function, posture and some limited tests. Look for the 'cascade' of normal finger posture, disrupted when flexor tendons are severed (Figure 8.1).

Fortunately in this age group most structures are flexible, so fractures are less likely. The biggest challenge is when there is a deep wound, which requires

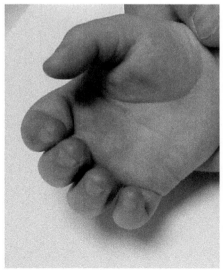

Figure 8.1 Normal finger cascade.

you to test the sensation and the tendons. You may need to explore the wound under local or general anaesthesia if still in doubt after examination.

Older children

Firstly, ask:

- If laceration present: Does your hand or your fingers feel funny or numb anywhere?

Look for:

- Deformity
- Swelling
- Distribution of lacerations

Test for:

- Range of movement of affected joints
- Localised tenderness (children can be remarkably specific if you test and retest, and get them to concentrate)
- Function of individual tendons
- Function of specific nerves
- Sensation

 Draw diagrams!

It is much easier to interpret written notes if diagrams are used. Most emergency departments have inkpads and body stamps.

Use the right terminology when writing notes.

- Avoid 'medial' and 'lateral' – use 'radial' and 'ulnar'.
- Avoid 'back' or 'front' or 'anterior' or 'posterior' – use 'dorsal' and 'volar' (or 'palmar'; see Figures 8.2 and 8.3).
- Do not number fingers (second, third, etc.); the digits are thumb, index, middle, ring and little.

Tendon examination

Remember that tendons also need testing in forearm wounds, as well as wounds of the hand itself.

Extensor tendons

Ask the child to bring their fingers out straight, and watch closely to make sure they can fully extend the fingers without any lag at any of the joints

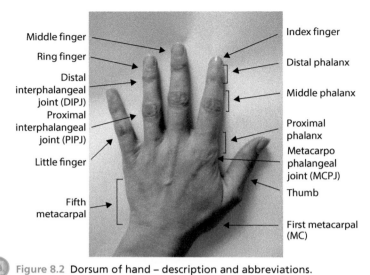

Middle finger

Ring finger

Distal interphalangeal joint (DIPJ)

Proximal interphalangeal joint (PIPJ)

Little finger

Fifth metacarpal

Index finger

Distal phalanx

Middle phalanx

Proximal phalanx

Metacarpo phalangeal joint (MCPJ)

Thumb

First metacarpal (MC)

Figure 8.2 Dorsum of hand – description and abbreviations.

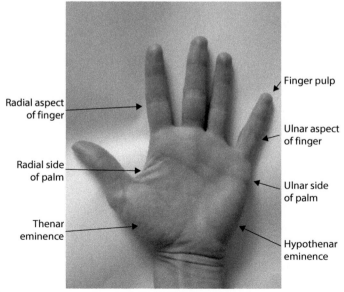

Radial aspect of finger

Radial side of palm

Thenar eminence

Finger pulp

Ulnar aspect of finger

Ulnar side of palm

Hypothenar eminence

Figure 8.3 Volar or palmar aspect of hand – descriptions.

(MCPJ, PIPJ and DIPJ). Remember that swelling or pain may sometimes prevent full extension. Next ask them to keep their fingers straight and not to let you bend the finger as you test each one's strength against resistance. Make this into a game, competing for strength. A finger with a partially severed tendon may look fully extended but there will be weakness and pain when resisting flexion.

Flexor tendons

There are two sets of flexor tendons. You need to understand the relationship of the two layers of tendons in order to understand the examination (Figure 8.4).

To test the superficial tendons, evaluate each individual finger in turn. Ask the child to place the hand, palm side up, on a flat surface. Then ask them to bend each finger, in turn, as you hold all the others down. The finger should flex at the MCPJ and PIPJ. Just like with extensor tendons, ask them to keep the finger there and not to let you straighten it, so you are also testing against resistance; if this is difficult there may be a partial tear.

To test the profundus tendons, again evaluate each individual finger in turn. Immobilise each finger against the flat surface, palm side up, by pressing down on the middle phalanx. Ask the child to bend the tip of the finger. The finger should flex at the DIPJ. Again test against resistance as we did above.

Video 8.1 Flexor and extensor tendon examination: https://youtu.be/LZ2q4ZO-SZM

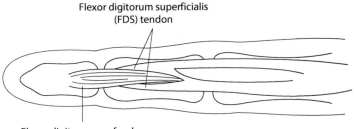

Flexor digitorum superficialis
(FDS) tendon

Flexor digitorum profundus
(FDP) tendon

Figure 8.4 Relationship of flexor tendons.

Nerve examination

Sensory function

Test for sensation by asking if light touch feels 'normal' or 'funny'. Do not ask the child simply if they can feel it, as sensation is rarely completely absent, and proprioception as well as some feeling will be present. If you think the child is not feeling normally and the area affected fits a nerve distribution pattern, you will need to refer to a hand specialist. Sometimes they say it is not normal, because it is swollen or painful. If this area is close to the injury and does not fit an anatomical pattern of a nerve, you do not need to worry.

The distribution of the sensory territories of the three major nerves may be quite variable. Damage to these large trunks occurs proximal to the wrist, so you need to check this with forearm or wrist wounds, and with fractures such as elbow fractures. For injuries of the hand itself, you will be testing the digital nerves. For the three main nerves, the most reliable places to test are the first web space for the radial nerve, the index fingertip for the median nerve and the little fingertip for the ulnar nerve (Figures 8.5 and 8.6). Far more commonly, the digital nerves are damaged. There are two main trunks for each digit, which run along the ulnar and radial sides dorsally, with equivalent palmar branches (see Figure 8.7). Again, absence of sensation is relative, not absolute.

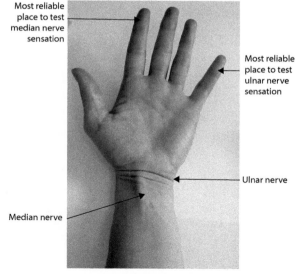

Figure 8.5 Location of median and ulnar nerves as they pass quite superficially through the wrist.

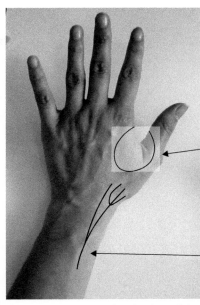

Most reliable place to test radial nerve sensation

Radial nerve

Figure 8.6 Path and distribution of the radial nerve.

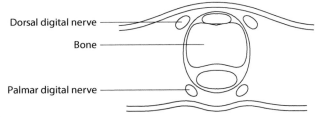

Dorsal digital nerve

Bone

Palmar digital nerve

Figure 8.7 Distribution of the digital nerves.

Motor function

If you are not sure if there is weakness, compare strength with the opposite hand. Weakness may also be caused by pain inhibiting the movement. This is where you need to be clear about your anatomy and therefore the risk of true nerve damage.

The radial nerve

The radial nerve supplies the wrist and finger and thumb extensors, which should be able to strongly resist flexion. Small children can be asked to give a 'thumbs up' sign.

The median nerve

The median nerve is best assessed by testing opposition. Ask the child to touch the tip of the thumb to the tip of the index finger, and to stop you 'breaking the ring'. Small children can be asked to give an 'OK' sign.

The ulnar nerve

The ulnar nerve operates most of the intrinsic muscles of the hand. A simple test is to put your pen between the child's little and ring fingers, and ask them to stop you pulling out. Small children can be asked to spread the fingers into a 'starfish' shape.

 Video 8.2 Radial, median and ulnar nerve examination: https://youtu.be/IASU3VgeZql

Wound exploration

Having reassured yourself that there is no damage to underlying structures by clinical examination, you should always confirm this by exploring any deep wound under local anaesthetic. Anything which glistens or looks white may be a tendon. Examine through the full range of movement, as severed tendons may retract and hide. Sometimes it can be difficult to assess a wound because of bleeding, and a tourniquet is required to create a bloodless field. In such cases, referral to a specialist is advised.

 Do not extend a wound in order to explore it!

 Seek advice if ever in doubt when exploring a hand wound!

FRACTURES OF THE HAND

There are some general rules which can be followed for phalangeal and metacarpal fractures:

- There should be a low threshold for ordering X-rays in hand injuries.
- Most injuries will cause swelling so the hand should be elevated in a high arm sling for a couple of days (see Chapter 15).

- Encourage exercises of the fingers.
- The best form of immobilisation is 'neighbour' or 'buddy' strapping (see Chapter 15), which allows movement in the inter-phalangeal joints (IPJs).
- If the neck or shaft of a metacarpal or phalanx is fractured, examine for finger rotation.

First, ask the child to lift the hand up to your eye level and check that the nails look reasonably aligned, and that the affected finger is not rotated (Figure 8.8a). Then ask them to drop their hand down, turn it the other way around and slowly open and close their fist (Figure 8.8b). Lastly, ensure you request the correct X-ray view (see Table 7.1 in Chapter 7). To see a finger clearly you need an antero-posterior and lateral view of the finger itself.

Rotation of the little finger (clinodactyly) is fairly common in normal people but is bilateral – compare the degree of rotation with the uninjured hand.

Video 8.3 Examining for finger rotation: https://youtu.be/hzaVyanzDeU

Metacarpal fractures
Assessment
The two main mechanisms are a punch (usually teenagers) or a fall onto the hand (less common). A glancing blow against an object does not generally cause a fracture. A fracture of the neck of the 5th metacarpal is often called a 'boxer's fracture'.

Examine carefully for rotational deformity (see the previous section). Check for a wound near the knuckles. You cannot tell if a wound communicates with the metacarpo-phalangeal joint, but it may, and will require a joint wash-out. Teenagers who punch inanimate objects are at low risk of infection, whereas if the wound has been caused by contact with another person's teeth there is a high risk of infection. Check the circumstances of the punch, and whether there are safeguarding or bullying issues.

X-ray
Both greenstick and growth plate injuries may occur. You will have requested a 'hand' view. Note that the views taken are usually an antero-posterior and an oblique view. If a displaced fracture is found (Figure 8.9), you may require a true lateral view to adequately assess displacement.

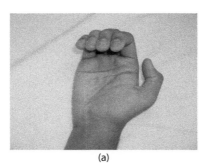

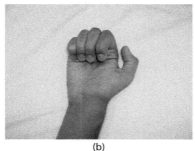

Figure 8.8 Assessment of finger rotation: (a) looking at nail alignment (normal), (b) looking at closure to fist (normal).

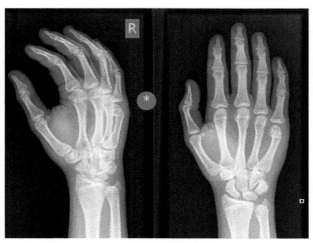

Figure 8.9 Fractured neck of the 5th metacarpal.

Management

Refer to the hand surgery service if there is rotational deformity, angulation greater than 20° in the metaphysis, angulation greater than 45° at the neck of the 5th metacarpal, more than 50% displacement of the bone ends, a potential open fracture or non-greenstick fractures in three adjacent metacarpals. For straightforward metacarpal fractures, apply neighbour strapping to the appropriate digit and elevate the hand in a high arm sling (see Chapter 15). Arrange hand specialist follow-up.

Fractures of the proximal and middle phalanges

Assessment

These fractures are commonly caused in ball games, but can be caused by a fall. Fracture patterns include transverse, spiral, epiphyseal and greenstick fractures. These can occur in the head, neck, shaft or base of the phalanx, or at the inter-phalangeal joints.

X-ray

Clinical discrimination between minor soft tissue injury and fractures is poor, and although only a small minority of fractures need operative intervention, these are important to detect in order to prevent long-term disability, so have a low threshold for X-ray.

Management

Refer to your hand surgery specialist if there is finger rotation, angulation greater than 20°, displacement of the bone ends (see Figure 8.10) or an intra-articular fracture. For uncomplicated fractures, neighbour strap the affected digit, place in a high arm sling (see Chapter 15) and arrange hand specialist follow-up.

Dislocations of the proximal and distal inter-phalangeal joints

Assessment

The PIPJ and the DIPJ can dislocate, either in a volar or a dorsal (more likely) direction, following hyper-flexion or hyper-extension injuries, usually in sports but sometimes due to a fall. Actual rupture of the collateral ligaments is rare compared with adults.

X-ray

Do not be fooled by the AP view, which may look normal, other than apparent loss of joint space. However in the lateral view dislocation is usually obvious (Figure 8.11). There may be an associated fracture.

Management

The joint needs to be reduced as soon as possible. Reduction usually requires a digital block (see Chapter 15) and you will get a better grip

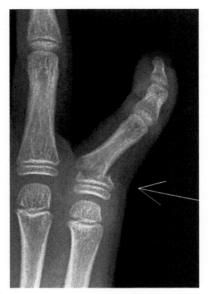

Figure 8.10 Displaced fracture base of proximal phalanx.

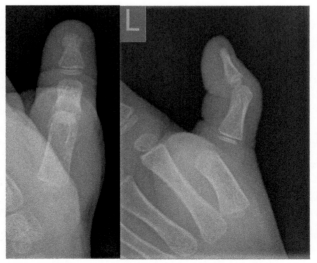

Figure 8.11 Dislocated thumb metacarpo-phalangeal joint.

if you wrap the distal finger in gauze. Holding the proximal bone tight, with your other hand tug gently on the distal part to disimpact it, then slide the joint back into position. Be relatively gentle, as compared with adults it is possible to overdo it and superimpose soft tissues into the joint. Following reduction take another X-ray to confirm, then neighbour strap to the next finger and elevate the hand. Refer for follow-up to your hand clinic.

 Video 8.4 Reduction of a dislocated finger: https://youtu.be/k8A2I53HMeg

Volar plate injury

This is an injury of the proximal inter-phalangeal joint on the volar side. It is caused by hyperextension, with the child often saying that the finger was 'bent back', usually in ball games. The complex 'volar plate' of the joint capsule pulls away from the volar surface of the base of the middle phalanx or it can pull off a fragment of bone of variable size.

X-ray

The X-ray findings are subtle and easily missed, unless a true lateral view of the finger is obtained and you look closely (Figure 8.12).

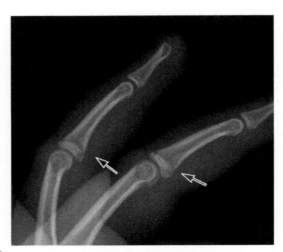

 Figure 8.12 Avulsion fractures of the volar plate at the proximal inter-phalangeal joints.

You need a 'finger' view with a true lateral to diagnose this injury; a 'hand' view does not give you the detail or the right view.

Management

If the fragment is large and contains a significant part of the articular surface it may need fixation. Fortunately, the fragment is usually small, especially in younger patients, and rarely needs surgical treatment, but opinion differs regarding immobilisation. Arrange hand clinic follow-up, to avoid a fixed flexion deformity of the PIPJ in the future.

Fractures of the distal phalanx

Assessment

These are usually sustained by crush injuries (Figure 8.13), and may involve more than one finger. Fractures of the distal phalanx are usually relatively unimportant injuries in themselves. Often there is associated skin or tissue loss, or nailbed damage (this is covered in 'Fingertip soft tissue injuries', later in this chapter).

X-ray

A fracture of the body of the distal phalanx is also called a 'tuft' fracture, or a fracture of the 'terminal' phalanx. Much less commonly, there may be a physeal injury. In this case (Figure 8.14a), the fracture was displaced. This required surgical fixation (Figure 8.14b).

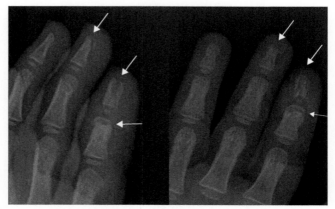

 Figure 8.13 Crush fractures of distal and middle phalanges.

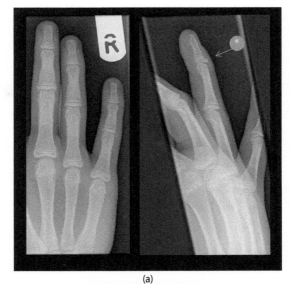

(a)

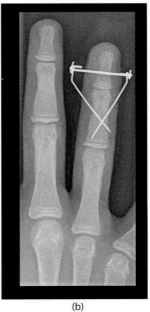

(b)

Figure 8.14 (a) Displaced Salter–Harris type III injury of the distal phalanx, (b) after surgical fixation.

Management

If there is no displacement, then neighbour strap the finger and arrange hand clinic follow-up. For displaced fractures involving the physis, consult with orthopaedics.

FINGERTIP SOFT TISSUE INJURIES

Fingertips are complex anatomical structures which are frequently injured (most often shut in closing doors). These crush injuries are very distressing to children and their families, so consider giving some intranasal opiate (see Chapter 2), to alleviate both pain and anxiety, and to make your examination easier. Confusingly, these injuries evoke widely differing opinions in their management. Unfortunately, robust, long-term outcome studies do not exist to assist you in your decisions.

General principles

The main principles of management are as follows:

- Children's fingertips are extremely good at regenerating themselves, so conservative management is possible in most cases, with a good cosmetic outcome.
- Restoration of normal anatomy is the aim; much can be achieved with adhesive strips, tissue glue and dressings; sutures are not usually needed.
- Long-term problems may occur at the base of the nail if the nail is avulsed and the nailfold is allowed to adhere onto the germinal matrix, resulting in abnormal growth of the new nail into the nailbed; this must be prevented (see 'Nail and nailbed injuries').
- Try to determine the presence or absence of a nailbed laceration; in many cases this is an educated guess.
- The presence of a subungual haematoma larger than 50% of the nail, or an underlying fracture, make a nailbed laceration more likely.

Nailbed injuries in children heal well. There is little evidence of improvement of outcome in repairing a nailbed laceration in children. Given that most such injuries require operative repair, most clinicians advocate only repairing the most obvious of injuries. Do not remove the nail in order to find out if there is one.

Assessment

It helps to think methodically about the different components of the fingertip:

- Is the injury still bleeding?
- Is it a dirty injury?
- Is it a nail or a pulp injury, or both?
- Is there any bone exposed?
- If proximal to the DIPJ, what is the level of the amputation?
- How damaged is the skin and is there skin missing?
- Is the nail is avulsed from its germinal matrix under the cuticle?
- Is there anatomical stability or will you need sutures to re-oppose wound edges?
- Is there a subungual haematoma? If so, is it able to ooze or is it contained and causing pain through pressure?

X-Ray

A typical X-ray would be the same as Figure 8.13.

Most crush injuries require an X-ray!

Management

This depends on findings on examination. Be methodical in your assessment; do not let the surrounding anxiety of the family (and sometimes staff) distract you, in order to consider putting in a digital block (see Chapter 15) for analgesia, and in order to allow you to properly examine the damage. Since the exact injuries are variable in structures affected and in dimensions, the principles outlined below will guide you. If there is an associated fracture, prescribe an antibiotic such as flucloxacillin and ensure follow-up is early (3–4 days). Always use non-adherent dressings, e.g. paraffin-impregnated gauze or a silicon-based dressing.

Persistent bleeding

Apply a non-adhesive dressing, bandage tightly, elevate in a high arm sling (see Chapter 15) and leave well alone for at least 20 minutes.

Tissue loss

If bone is exposed, or the skin is very contused, contaminated or non-viable, refer to a hand specialist. The exception is the pulp itself, which has excellent powers of regeneration even if there is a considerable amount missing. For injuries proximal to the DIPJ, every attempt should be made to preserve the amputated part. It should be covered with sterile, soaked dressings, sealed in a plastic bag, and placed within another bag containing ice. The remaining finger should be covered with a non-adherent dressing, and elevated in a high arm sling.

If referral is not needed, use non-adhesive dressings, and bandage the area to stay clean and dry (see Chapter 15 for how to achieve this in small children). Ideally it should be left in peace for 5 days before review, as constant disturbance slows healing.

Nail and nailbed injuries

This is a controversial area and there is no good evidence that a perfectionist approach is needed in children (see general principles, above). Nails grow from the base (Figure 8.15). If the nail base has popped out from under the cuticle, the underlying germinal matrix is likely to be disrupted, and if the gap is allowed to close, normal longitudinal growth of the new nail may not occur. Similarly, a large nailbed laceration will affect the growth of the new nail. Not only will the defect be cosmetic, but it may be painful.

If the nail is very loose, remove the nail and inspect the nailbed, and repair with fine sutures if needed. If the nail is quite firmly adherent, attempts should not be made to remove it as this causes further damage. Seek advice.

If the nail has already been avulsed or you have had to remove it, it should be replaced back in the nailfold (Figure 8.16). Various techniques can be employed. First clean the nail and trim any attached skin. If the nail is lost, a substitute splint must be inserted. This may be custom made using the wax paper backing of paraffin gauze dressings. Once in position, a combination of tissue glue across the nailfold with adhesive strips over the fingertip is usually sufficient to keep it in place for a week or two. Sometimes a suture either side ('stay' sutures) may be needed.

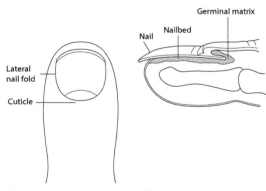

Figure 8.15 The nail and nailbed.

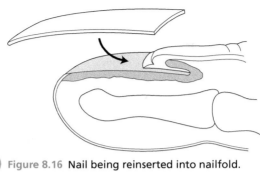

Figure 8.16 Nail being reinserted into nailfold.

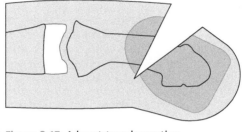

Figure 8.17 A burst-type laceration.

If the base of the nail is still inserted into the nailfold under the cuticle, the nail is best left alone even if there is a deep laceration through it. To repair an underlying nailbed injury would require removal of the nail and risking further harm, whereas these distal nail injuries do well with conservative management.

Anatomically unstable injuries

Large burst-type lacerations (Figure 8.17) or those involving more than 50% of the digital circumference are likely to be anatomically unstable and require sutures. Milder lacerations can usually be maintained with adhesive strips and a supportive dressing. Just try bringing the tissues back into alignment and see if adhesive strips and glue will suffice – usually they will. If the wound edges are ragged and do not oppose well, do not worry – children heal well and the gaps will fill in quickly.

If suturing through nail is required, this can be quite difficult. One suture each side can be taken first through the nail, then through the skin (usually in two steps), and then each side can then be pulled tight, bringing the nail into position symmetrically.

Subungual haematoma

Crush injuries to fingertips may cause a subungual haematoma. This is a collection of blood underneath the nail because the nailbed has torn but the overlying nail has remained intact. The blood under the nail may escape out of the side of the nail, but often becomes trapped underneath, causing pressure to build up in this very sensitive area. Trephining the nail releases the blood and is a very satisfying procedure because of the instant relief of symptoms (see Chapter 15). It is not uncommon for subungual haematoma to present 24 hours or so after injury. If the haematoma is large enough to be causing pain, it is worth trephining – the central area is often liquid and you will achieve symptomatic relief.

Underlying fracture

For all except minor fingertip injuries, an X-ray should be performed. If a fracture is present, but confined to the shaft of the distal phalanx and undisplaced, a simple dressing may be applied and oral flucloxacillin prescribed if the skin is broken. If the fracture is through the epiphyseal plate, or the base of the distal phalanx is displaced, refer to a specialist.

TENDON AND NERVE INJURIES

See 'Clinical examination' at the top of the chapter for assessment.

Management

All suspected injuries should be referred the same day to your hand service.

OTHER SOFT TISSUE FINGER INJURIES

Ulnar collateral ligament injury

This is an unusual injury which affects the base of the thumb at the 1st metacarpo-phalangeal joint. In adults, a true rupture of the ulnar collateral ligament (UCL) occurs, but in children it is associated with a Salter–Harris III fracture of the base of the proximal phalanx and the UCL itself is intact. It happens with forced abduction of the thumb.

Management

All suspected injuries should be referred immediately to your hand service.

Mallet finger

This is also an unusual injury. A true mallet finger is the rupture of the extensor tendon as it inserts onto the distal phalanx. This is fairly common in adults, and can occur in teenagers. In younger children, as in a UCL injury, it is more likely to be associated with an avulsion fracture of the physis and the actual tendon is intact. There is obvious droop of the distal phalanx when you look at it side-on.

Management

Immobilise with the digit in slight hyperextension in a splint and refer to a hand clinic. The splint must not be removed until review. At that point the hand specialists may allow removal to clean the finger and let the skin 'breathe' but it is crucial that the joint is not flexed while free, as the tendon is very slow to heal.

Mallet splints are available, made out of plastic, but the skin sweats and becomes a little macerated under these. Zimmer splints (aluminium with foam backing) are preferable, and can be custom made to cover the dorsum of the digit, curving round to incorporate the DIPJ, keeping the DIPJ in slight extension. Zimmer splints are less robust, so possibly more suitable for adults than children. There are pros and cons to both – follow your local policy.

 Video 8.5 Application of mallet splint: https://youtu.be/ZDSvVWaqhrY

INFECTIONS

Paronychia

This is a localised infection, usually around the cuticle. It is usually caused by nail-biting. Once the infection has progressed from the reddened stage to develop a collection of pus, antibiotics are useless and drainage is required.

Management

Incision and drainage is required once pus has formed. A digital block may be needed (see Chapter 15). If a large collection of pus is visible this may not be necessary as the overlying skin is dead. Insert a scalpel blade directly into the pus, making a decent sized hole, then 'milk' the finger to extrude all pus. Cover with a non-adherent dressing, and advise the family to soak the finger in warm water twice over the next 24 hours, milking any remaining pus out themselves. If a paronychia is persistent more than 10 days, consider the presence of underlying osteomyelitis, and request an X-ray.

Tendon infection

Any wound infection may cause tendon infection. Flexor tendons are contained within synovial sheaths, and infection can spread rapidly and be extremely destructive. The signs of this are pain, especially on finger extension, with erythema and generalised (fusiform) swelling. The child will be holding the finger in a slightly flexed position. This condition requires urgent referral.

Refer immediately to a hand specialist if you have any suspicion of flexor tendon infection!

Pulp and palmar space infections

A collection of pus in the pulp space of the fingertip is called a felon. The finger pulp is hot, red, swollen, fluctuant and extremely painful. Refer to a hand specialist for surgical treatment. The palm contains soft tissue spaces, confined by fascial compartments. If infection occurs, signs may be subtle because the infection is deep seated. Look for the loss of the normal dip between the metacarpals, and test for pain on compression.

Refer immediately to a hand specialist if you have any suspicion of flexor tendon infection!

CUT WRISTS IN DELIBERATE SELF-HARM

Unfortunately deliberate self-harm (DSH) involving forearm or wrist cutting has become fairly common in teenagers in the UK and other countries. It is a sign of psychological distress, which may merit referral to a mental health specialist. The child may or may not be forthcoming that a wound was caused by DSH.

Suspect deliberate self-harm if you ever see superficial lacerations on the insides of the wrists!

REFLEX SYMPATHETIC DYSTROPHY/COMPLEX REGIONAL PAIN SYNDROME

This is a dysautonomia which occurs from the age of 8 or so. It usually follows injury, and can cause chronic debilitating wasting of the arm or leg. Emergency physicians tend to see milder versions soon after injury, and in fact there can be dysautonomia immediately after injury. It can present quite dramatically with pallor, coldness, hyperaesthesia or swelling or stiffness of a limb, commonly the forearm and hand. Milder autonomic nervous system symptoms occur temporarily quite frequently in teenage girls with hand or ankle injuries and can be mistaken for fractures or dislocations with vascular injury. There may be a very abnormal posture, but the overriding feature is severe pain, even to light touch.

Without early intervention symptoms tend to worsen. Delay in diagnosis is common, and frequently follows multiple radiological imaging due to clinical concern about a missed injury because of the degree of pain, and prolonged immobilisation in an attempt to treat the pain, which only makes things worse since the symptoms will resolve with normal use of the limb.

Management

Reassure the patient and parent that there is no severe injury. Be sympathetic and patient, but try to get the affected part to move to demonstrate that there is not a major mechanical issue. This may need passive demonstration of movements, or getting the child to achieve one or two small movements.

Give the patient and parents a goal-orientated, staged physiotherapy programme, involving increasing mobilisation each day for the next 7–14 days. Very small goals each day, which increase the mobility, must be set. Encourage a positive outlook and convey the idea that the child should be back to normal in 7–14 days. Avoid immobilising the affected part (e.g. splints, plaster, crutches). Do not discharge without arranging follow-up by someone experienced in these problems. If things are not improving at 14 days, formal physiotherapy, possibly with psychological input, is needed. In most cases, particularly if the parent understands the exercise programme and is prepared to encourage the child, things will be fine by 2 weeks post-injury.

THE LOWER LIMB

INTRODUCTION

You will see that this chapter has a heavy emphasis on 'the limping child'. This is because children can limp from a serious non-traumatic cause, but may present with a vague history of trauma as their carers try to attribute a cause for the limp. Furthermore, minor trauma can expose underlying pathology (such as a slipped epiphysis or bone tumour). For this reason, non-traumatic conditions are included later in this chapter.

Consider non-traumatic causes for limping in children, even if a history of trauma is offered!

INJURIES OF THE HIP AND FEMUR

Avulsion fractures around the hip

Children may sustain avulsion fractures following sudden movements, usually during sport. The five places this can occur are the ischial tuberosity, the greater and lesser trochanters of the femur and the anterior superior and anterior inferior iliac spine (Figures 9.1 through 9.4). The clue is in the history. The child may or may not be able to weight-bear. X-ray if you get the right mechanism of injury and the child can localise the pain. Although most are managed conservatively unless significant displacement is present, a diagnosis helps you to give cautious discharge advice, such as staying off sports for 6 weeks. Refer to orthopaedics for follow-up.

The same five apophyses can become inflamed with repetitive sports use, rather than fracture acutely. Other traction apophysitis conditions include Osgood–Schlatter disease of the knee (see 'Other injuries of the knee') and Sever's disease of the heel (see 'Other heel problems').

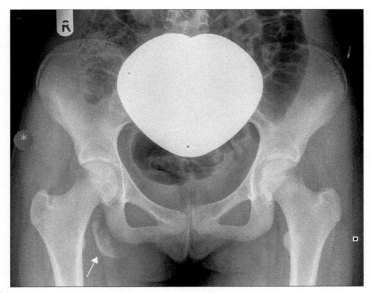

Figure 9.1 Avulsion fracture of the right ischial tuberosity.

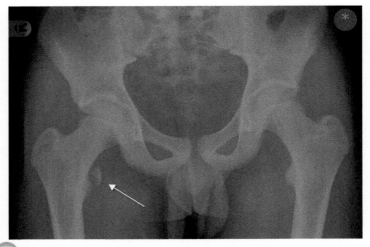

Figure 9.2 Avulsion fracture of the right lesser trochanter.

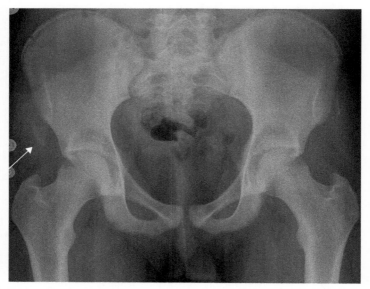

Figure 9.3 Avulsion fracture of the right anterior superior iliac spine.

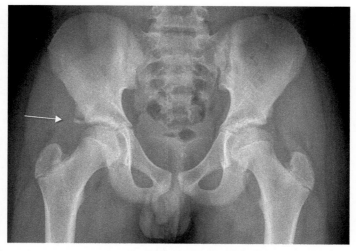

Figure 9.4 Avulsion fracture of the right anterior inferior iliac spine.

Femoral shaft fractures

Considerable force is usually required to fracture the femur. There is usually a history of a fall with the leg twisted awkwardly under the child. Femoral shaft fractures alone can be responsible for significant bleeding, although in isolation will not cause clinical signs of shock.

Assess A B C and check for other injuries!
Does the history fit? (Is it a non-accidental injury?)

Assessment

Diagnosis is usually obvious. There is significant swelling of the affected thigh, and it is painful to move. The child will be unable to weight-bear or lift the limb off the bed, and will be in considerable pain. In infants and toddlers with chubby thighs, signs are more subtle.

X-ray

Fractures may be transverse, spiral (Figure 9.5) or supracondylar. Seventy percent occur in the middle third of the femur. You must be able to see the joint above and below the fracture on the image, to screen for associated injuries such as metaphyseal fractures (see Chapter 14, Non-Accidental Injury).

Management

Support the leg with something like a blanket, with the hip and knee slightly flexed. The child will require intra-nasal or intravenous opiate

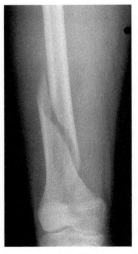

Figure 9.5 Spiral fracture of the femur.

analgesia and a femoral nerve block (see Chapters 2 and 15), ideally before moving to X-ray and receiving definitive splintage.

Following radiographic confirmation, refer to an orthopaedic surgeon for admission to hospital. Younger children will be placed in traction (Gallows' for infants, skin traction for older children), sometimes followed by a spica plaster cast. The over 5s may be considered for an intramedullary nail.

INJURIES OF THE KNEE

It is important to remember that knee pain is sometimes the result of hip joint pathology and clinical examination of the hip should always be undertaken.

 Slipped upper femoral epiphysis (SUFE) may present with isolated thigh or knee pain!

Most acute knee injuries are sprains, sustained during sport or while falling over, usually with a history of twisting. Major fractures and meniscal or ligamentous tears are uncommon in children under 12 years.

Avulsion fractures of the tibial spine occur in younger children and teenagers, and can be quite subtle; they are the equivalent of an anterior cruciate ligament injury in adults. As we see in the ulnar collateral ligament of the thumb or avulsion injuries in children elsewhere, such as around the hip or knee, the bone where ligaments and tendon attach is often more vulnerable than the more elastic ligament or tendon. Thus, avulsion injuries often occur in children, in circumstances where a ligament or tendon rupture might occur in an adult.

Acute knee injuries

Assessment
Accurate assessment of acute knee injuries can be difficult because of pain. Your notes should record if the patient is fully, partially or non-weight-bearing, and the range of movement of the joint (from 0° to 120°). After injury the knee is often held flexed and will not extend. This is referred to as a 'locked' knee. In adults locking is suggestive of a meniscal injury or a loose fragment of bone within the joint, but in children hamstring spasm is often the primary cause of the inability to extend the knee. It can usually be overcome with gentle persuasion by putting your hand under the knee, on the couch, and asking the child just to touch it with

the back of their knee, if only for a second, just to prove they can do it. You may need Entonox® analgesia to relax the child. Persistent hamstring spasm precludes any reliable examination. Examination should include assessment of the joint, the ligaments and the extensor mechanism.

The joint

An effusion is the cardinal sign of an injury within the joint. It is most easily identified with the knee extended but this is not always possible. In a similar way as the elbow, compare with the opposite side to detect a subtle effusion. By and large if there is no effusion, serious injury is unlikely. A large effusion that develops within less than an hour of the injury usually consists of blood (a haemarthrosis) and indicates significant intra-articular injury – usually a fracture or a significant ligament or joint capsule tear.

The ligaments

Ligament injury is best assessed with the knee in a slightly flexed position. To achieve this, the child needs to relax, which is difficult when they are in pain. The optimum way to achieve this is as follows: Bend your own knee and put it under the child's, so that the child's leg is slightly bent and supported on your thigh. Getting the child to relax their leg on yours may take a little encouragement.

First palpate to see if there is focal tenderness and then check that the ligaments are intact. When assessing if a ligament is intact, remember that children are stretchy. Assess the normal side first to see how stretchy it is, and to gain the child's confidence.

The medial collateral runs from the medial femoral condyle to the medial aspect of the tibia; the lateral collateral runs from the lateral femoral condyle to the fibula. After palpation, gently stress the ligaments by resting one of your hands on the thigh to check it is relaxed, then holding the child's lower leg in your other hand and exerting a valgus and varus strain.

To assess the cruciate ligaments, flex the knee to 90° and gently sit yourself on the child's toes. Grasp the upper tibia with both hands and push and pull it back and forth to test for laxity. You may need to compare with their unaffected side.

The extensor mechanism

The extensor mechanism consists of the quadriceps muscle, the patella, the patella tendon and the tibial tuberosity. Injury can disrupt these

Video 9.1 Knee examination: https://youtu.be/Xetl69SWUGE

components at their junctions with each other. You should therefore palpate along this anatomy to identify any localised tenderness, gap or swelling. Then see if the child can actively extend their knee by getting them to do a 'straight leg raise'. This means raising the whole leg up, with the knee in full extension and toes dorsi-flexed towards the body, so that the heel lifts off the examination couch.

X-ray

X-ray if the child is completely non-weight-bearing, if there is a large effusion, or if the mechanism of injury is significant. The Ottawa knee rules can apply from puberty.

The Ottawa rules reduce the need to X-ray. Only X-ray children over 12 years old if:

- The child is/was unable to weight-bear two steps on the affected side both at the time of injury and now – this may need a little coaxing in order to prevent unnecessary X-rays
- There is tenderness at the neck of the fibula
- There is tenderness over the patella
- The child is unable to flex to 90°

Small osteochondral fractures avulsed from the surface of the joint are easily overlooked but are important to detect (Figure 9.6). If you cannot see a fracture, ensure you are not missing one by checking for radiographic

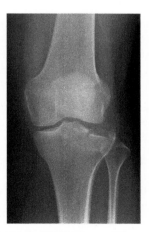

 Figure 9.6 Fracture of the tibial plateau.

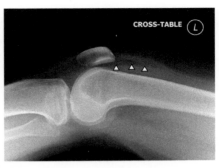

 Figure 9.7 Lipohaemarthrosis of the knee.

 You can see that behind the patella there is a black, lucent shadow which contains a fluid level (remember that the leg has been placed horizontally).

signs of an effusion as we did with the fat pads in the elbow (see Chapter 7). An effusion, haemarthrosis or lipohaemarthrosis (Figure 9.7) can be seen on the lateral view and are clues that you should ensure orthopaedic follow-up for your patient.

Management

If you see a fracture, it is best to refer for same-day orthopaedic consultation. Otherwise, all other injuries can be reviewed in an orthopaedic clinic, ideally a week or so later, when the pain and swelling are decreasing. There is little evidence for compression bandages, which soon loosen beyond usefulness, but a splint such as a detachable 'cricket pad splint' can be very useful, used with crutches. Advise elevation when not walking around, and encourage quadriceps exercises to prevent muscle wasting; this is simply repetitive straight leg raises, aiming for 50 a day!

Patellar fracture

Fractures of the patella can be caused by a direct trauma but are rare in childhood. Osteochondral fractures of the patella are most often caused during patella dislocation/relocation. Children can also sustain a 'sleeve' fracture, which occurs on sudden quadriceps contraction, such as jumping. The inferior pole of the patella is avulsed. The bony fragment sometimes looks trivial on X-rays but there is often a large chunk of articular cartilage attached to it and the injury is significant.

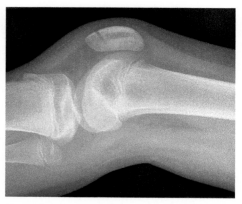

 Figure 9.8 Fracture of the body of the patella.

Assessment

There will be pain and swelling around the patella and difficulty extending the knee or performing a straight leg raise (see 'Assessment' section in 'Acute knee injuries').

X-ray

There are four types of image you may see. First is a true fracture of the body of the patella (Figure 9.8); second is a congenital bipartite patella, which may be mistaken for a fracture; third is the patellar sleeve fracture (Figure 9.9), which is the most difficult to spot; and lastly, a patellar dislocation can cause a small fracture (see 'Patellar dislocation'). A congenital bipartite patella occurs when there is an accessory bone found in the upper, outer quadrant of the patella. The edges are rounded, and there are no matching clinical signs.

Management

Refer immediately to orthopaedics if you suspect a fracture.

Patellar dislocation

Assessment

This often follows a direct blow to the medial side of the knee, but may happen spontaneously, for example twisting while running. It is most frequently seen in adolescent girls and is often recurrent. On examination, the patient usually holds the knee in flexion, with obvious lateral displacement of the patella.

X-ray

If the mechanism of injury does not imply severe force, you can reduce this dislocation before imaging. Following reduction, X-rays are mandatory to check for a small osteochondral fracture of the articular surface, either at

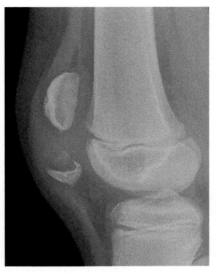

 Figure 9.9 Patellar sleeve fracture.

 A patellar sleeve fracture may look small and innocent on the X-ray but there will be significant disruption to the articular cartilage.
Note the high-riding patella, the avulsed crescent-shaped fragment and localised swelling around the lower pole of the patella. There is typically no joint effusion as this is an extra-articular fracture.

the back of the patella or over the lateral femoral condyle, sustained either during dislocation or reduction. A 'skyline' view may be needed but may be impossible as it requires the knee to be flexed, and at this stage there is often a haemarthrosis and too much pain; it can be done at follow-up instead.

Management
Do not obtain an X-ray to confirm dislocation – this is very obvious clinically. Go straight to reduction. Reduction of a dislocated patella can often be achieved using Entonox® for analgesic and sedative effect. Entonox® should be inhaled for 1–2 minutes prior to attempting reduction of the dislocation. Reduction is often achieved spontaneously as the patient is encouraged to relax the quadriceps, to allow the knee to slowly extend. Reduction can be assisted with firm, but gentle pressure over the lateral aspect of the patella, using both of your thumbs, while an assistant simultaneously helps to gently extend the knee by holding the heel. After

the patella is reduced, apply a full-length cylinder plaster or splint ('cricket' splint), and arrange orthopaedic clinic follow-up.

Other injuries of the knee

Other problems of the knee related to repeated usage and minor trauma of the knee can include Osgood–Schlatter disease, Sinding-Larsen-Johansson syndrome and osteochondritis dissecans.

Assessment

Osgood–Schlatter disease (Figure 9.10) is a traction apophysitis of the patellar tendon as it inserts into the tibial tuberosity, particularly

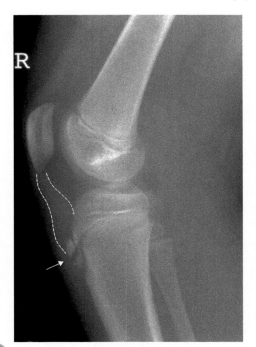

 Figure 9.10 Osgood–Schlatter disease.

 Osgood–Schlatter disease is primarily a clinical diagnosis. Fragmentation of the tibial tuberosity (arrow in Figure 9.10) is common in normal teenagers but swelling of the patellar tendon and blurring of the fat planes does suggest local inflammation. The dotted lines demonstrate swelling of the patellar tendon.

common in sporty children during late childhood and early adolescence. It is bilateral in about a quarter of cases and often takes up to 18 months to resolve. Localised pain is felt at the tibial tuberosity, and symptoms are worse following activity and improve with rest. On examination a lump is seen or felt around the tibial tuberosity, due to microfractures and subsequent callus formation. The lump may be tender.

Sinding-Larsen-Johansson syndrome is less common but gives rise to similar symptoms at the other end of the patella tendon where it joins the lower pole of the patella. Osteochondritis dissecans (Figure 9.11) is another disease which presents with knee pain. Cracks in the articular cartilage and underlying subchondral bone over time cause pain and swelling, knee locking and a crackling sound with joint movement. These diseases are not caused by a single episode of trauma, but are mentioned because an injury may provoke a consultation for the more chronic condition.

X-ray
X-rays are not necessary if the clinical picture is characteristic.

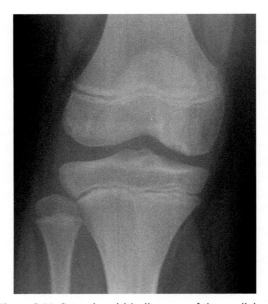

 Figure 9.11 Osteochondritis dissecans of the medial femoral condyle.

Management

The child should be advised to reduce their level of activity according to the pain. This is a difficult trade-off and some will continue normal sports; this is not harmful. Reassurance that this is a common condition is often sufficient. Persistent difficulties in doing sports may respond to physiotherapy, and rarely a plaster cast may be needed. Management should be led by an orthopaedic specialist.

Fractures of the tibia and fibula

Assessment

Fractures of the lateral malleolus are more common, but less so than in adults. Greenstick-type fractures can occur. Fractures of the shaft of either the tibia or fibula usually require significant trauma and are uncommon in children. The exception to this, and the commonest fracture, is called a 'toddler's fracture' and is seen in ambulant 1- to 3-year-olds, when minor twisting trauma can result in spiral fracture. It can even occur on suddenly standing up. Unlike other long-bone spiral fractures (femur and humerus), toddler's fractures are not usually suspicious of non-accidental injury.

On examining for a toddler's fracture, findings are subtle. There is no swelling, and direct pressure often does not often elicit tenderness. The clue is in twisting the foot with dorsiflexion. This causes torsion of the tibia, which moves the fracture and causes pain.

X-ray

As in the forearm, greenstick fractures can occur in the tibia and fibula (Figure 9.12).

The diagnosis may be obvious, but greenstick fractures and toddler's fractures can be subtle (see Figure 9.14). In a toddler's fracture the periosteum can hold the bone so tightly that displacement does not occur, and there may be no visible X-ray changes. However, around 10 days later, reabsorption along the fracture line and callus at the outer cortex are visible. In Figure 9.13 the fracture is visible in both views, if you look carefully. Figure 9.14 shows a fracture in the healing phase, showing periosteal reaction.

Management

Undisplaced greenstick fractures and toddler's fractures may be immobilised in an above-knee plaster cast. For all other fractures obtain an orthopaedic

If you suspect a toddler's fracture and the X-ray is normal, treat as fractured and review in 10 days!

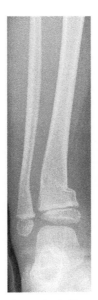

Figure 9.12 Greenstick
fracture of the distal tibia.

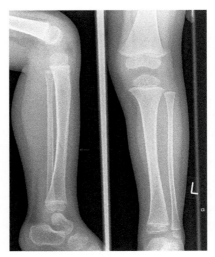

Figure 9.13 Spiral fracture of the tibia
('toddler's fracture').

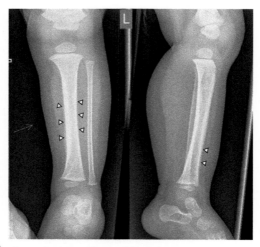

 Figure 9.14 Healing toddler's fracture.

 The arrows highlight periosteal thickening, seen as another line outlining the cortex on both sides.

opinion. If you suspect a toddler's fracture and cannot see it on the X-ray, immobilise the leg in an above-knee plaster and re-X-ray after 10 days.

ANKLE INJURIES

General procedures

Assessment

Ankle fractures are less common in children than adults, and if present, tend to be greenstick or epiphyseal fractures. As with other joints in children, an avulsion fracture is more likely than a ligament tear or sprain. Teenagers also present with a special category of fracture called 'transitional fractures' because they are in transition from adolescence to maturity. They sometimes appear innocuous but often involve the articular surface and require CT evaluation and surgical treatment. There are two common patterns: the Tillaux fracture and the triplane fracture. Use the Salter–Harris classification (Chapter 6, Figure 6.5) to alert you.

The well-known 'Ottawa ankle rules' for imaging in adult injuries apply to children aged 8 years and older. For younger children, bony tenderness or inability to weight-bear are indications for X-ray.

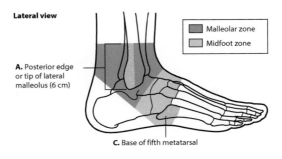

Lateral view

Malleolar zone
Midfoot zone

A. Posterior edge or tip of lateral malleolus (6 cm)

C. Base of fifth metatarsal

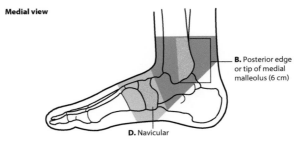

Medial view

B. Posterior edge or tip of medial malleolus (6 cm)

D. Navicular

Figure 9.15 Ottawa ankle rules illustration.

The Ottawa rules reduce the need to X-ray. Only X-ray children over 8 years old if:

- The child is/was unable to weight-bear two steps on the affected side both at the time of injury and now – this may need a little coaxing in order to prevent unnecessary X-rays
- There is tenderness at the tip or the posterior half of the lateral or medial malleolus (up to 6 cm from the tip)

When you examine and record your findings, you must be clear if there is medial and/or lateral tenderness, and whether each of these is bony or over the medial ligament complex (deltoid) or lateral ligament complex (usually the anterior talo-fibular ligament). Bilateral tenderness may imply an unstable ankle.

X-ray

Look for small avulsion fractures of the lateral malleolus, which are the commonest fracture pattern. In larger fractures it is important to look for signs of instability by checking that the gap between the talus and tibia and fibula is parallel, as it is when stable. In Figure 9.16 you can see that the gap between the talus and the articular surfaces of the tibia and fibula measures the same

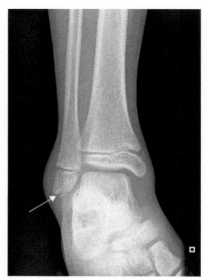

 Figure 9.16 Avulsion fracture of the lateral malleolus with normal joint congruity.

all the way around. This view is called a mortise view, and is a modified AP view to help you assess the joint congruity. Disruption of the articular surfaces or ligaments will result in movement called 'talar shift'. Medial malleolus fractures are less common and tend to be bigger (Figure 9.17).

Watch out for growth plate fractures involving the distal tibia. Fractures that extend into the articular surface can be easily overlooked on plain films and often need CT evaluation. This is especially true in the teenager who is vulnerable to transitional fractures (see above).

Management

Sprains can be treated in the usual way (see Chapter 3). Most children do not want or need to rest the ankle, but elevation to reduce swelling can help. The important thing about ligamentous injuries in the ankle is the loss of proprioception (balance). This is subtle, but if not recognised and the child returns to sports as soon as the bruising and swelling settles, the poor proprioception can make them re-injure the ankle easily.

Get the child to stand on one leg and they will see how wobbly the affected side is compared with the other leg. They should practice

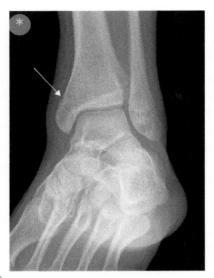

 Figure 9.17 **Medial malleolus fracture.**

balancing on one foot several times a day, for example when brushing teeth, practicing on the bottom stair and when more confident, standing on their bed or a football.

Children recover from sprains quickly and the use of crutches should be discouraged. The ankle can be regarded as healed once the proprioception and gait are normal. Referral for physiotherapy is beneficial for sporty children and re-injuries. Teenagers may take up to 6 weeks to recover. Follow-up appointments are not necessary, unless they are very hesitant to try mobilisation, in which case you should arrange physiotherapy or medical review to prevent complications (see Chapter 8 on regional complex pain syndrome).

If you see a fracture, refer immediately to orthopaedics if there is any talar shift, a displaced fragment or a fracture involving the articular surface, such as transitional fractures, which require internal fixation. For simple, undisplaced fractures, apply a below-knee backslab and arrange orthopaedic clinic follow-up. Small avulsion fractures can be treated as a sprain.

Calcaneum fracture

Assessment

The commonest cause of a calcaneal fracture is a fall from a height, usually higher than the child's head, and is unusual below 10 years old. There is

STOP Always assess the spine and pelvis for associated injury!

swelling and weight-bearing is very painful. The axial load exerted during injury can also cause lumbar spine and pelvic fractures. Stress fractures of the calcaneum can also occur (see 'Other heel problems').

X-ray

It is important to specifically request calcaneal views, as a normal AP and lateral of the foot may not reveal a calcaneal fracture (Figure 9.18). On the lateral view, do not confuse the calcaneal apophysis with a fracture. The fracture can be difficult to spot on the lateral view, but is crucial not to miss.

Bohler's angle will help you spot a fracture. Draw a horizontal line across the top of the calcaneum from its articulating point with the talus back to its tuberosity at the back. Now draw another line from the same articulating point with the talus forwards and down to the anterior articulating point. This angle should measure more than 20°. In Figure 9.19, Bohler's angle measures 26° and you can see a subtle fracture dividing the calcaneum in two. This fracture is not depressed so Bohler's angle is normal.

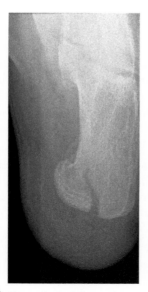

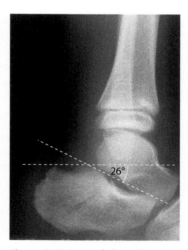

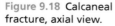 Figure 9.18 Calcaneal fracture, axial view.

Figure 9.19 Lateral view. Non depressed calcaneal fracture with a Bohler's angle in the normal range.

Management

Refer immediately to orthopaedics in case further imaging (CT) or admission for analgesia and elevation is needed.

Double check there are not bilateral calcaneal fractures; this is common and the pain from the worse side distracts patients and clinicians!

Other heel problems

Children may also get Achilles tendinitis, retrocalcaneal and Achilles bursitis, plantar fasciitis, calcaneal bursitis, calcaneal stress fractures and Sever's disease. Sever's disease is a traction apophysitis of the Achilles tendon where it inserts onto the calcaneum, similar to Osgood–Schlatter disease. It does not produce a lump like Osgood–Schlatter disease, affects a younger age group (8–13 years) and results in normal X-rays.

Treatment of all of these disorders is largely conservative. Do not worry if you cannot make a precise diagnosis – recommend non-steroidal anti-inflammatory medication and arrange orthopaedic follow-up.

INJURIES OF THE FEET

Fracture of the proximal 5th metatarsal

Assessment

These are usually caused by an inversion injury, causing peroneus brevis to avulse its bony attachment. On examination there is usually localised tenderness.

X-ray

Do not mistake the epiphysis, which lies parallel to the shaft of the 5th metatarsal, for a fracture. The apophysis itself may be avulsed or fractured (Figure 9.20). If in doubt, the exact site of tenderness should answer the question whether this is a normal epiphysis or an acute injury.

Management

Undisplaced fractures can be managed either in a below-knee backslab or

Most fractures are transverse, not longitudinal.

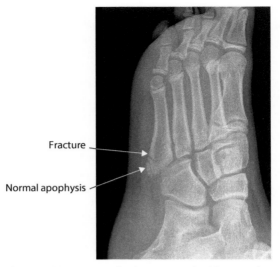

Fracture

Normal apophysis

 Figure 9.20 Fracture of 5th metatarsal with normal apophysis.

not immobilised and just supported by crutches, depending on ability to weight-bear and patient preference. Arrange orthopaedic clinic follow-up.

Other metatarsal injuries

Greenstick fractures of one or more metatarsals occur in small children when jumping from a height. Older children may sustain greenstick, epiphyseal, transverse neck fractures or spiral shaft fractures. Stress fractures may occur in athletic children. For multiple or displaced fractures, apply a below-knee plaster cast. Otherwise apply a crepe bandage and supply crutches. Arrange orthopaedic clinic follow-up.

Toe injuries

Assessment

Stubbed and crushed toes are common. Dislocations are unusual in children.

X-ray

Management is the same whether bruised or fractured, so X-rays are unnecessary unless involvement of the metatarsal is suspected.

Management

Treatment of crush and nail injuries is similar to fingertip injuries (see Chapter 8), although even more conservative. Dislocations can be reduced under a digital block (see Chapter 15). Otherwise, management is tricky because of pain and footwear issues; it consists of commonsense measures such as elevation, crutches and wide-fitting shoes. Neighbour strapping (see Chapter 15) may be of benefit after the initial swelling subsides. Show the family how to do it and allow them to take home some gauze and tape to try.

THE LIMPING CHILD

Limping in children is a common presentation. There may be no history of trauma, but sometimes minor injuries are recollected and the limp falsely attributed to an event in the previous few days. Hip joint pathology is common and may present with knee pain. Subtle restriction of hip internal rotation is the most sensitive clinical sign of hip joint pathology and should always be evaluated regardless of the site of pain.

 Hip pathology often presents as knee pain.

The differential diagnosis of limp is wide and includes septic arthritis, transient synovitis, Perthes disease, slipped upper femoral epiphysis (SUFE), inflammatory arthritides such as juvenile idiopathic arthritis, idiopathic chondrolysis, fractures, sprains and bone cancer. SUFE and septic arthritis deserve special mention, because diagnosis is often delayed or overlooked, and this can lead to serious long-term consequences for the patient.

The age of the child helps to determine the most likely diagnosis but there is overlap:

- 0-5: Septic arthritis, transient synovitis, Perthes disease
- 5-10: Transient synovitis, septic arthritis, Perthes disease, SUFE
- 10-15: SUFE, transient synovitis, Perthes disease, septic arthritis

Investigation depends on your local policy, and depends on the severity of symptoms and risk of other pathology. Investigations may include X-ray, ultrasound, white count, C-reactive protein and erythrocyte sedimentation rate.

Transient synovitis

This is a harmless temporary inflammation of the synovium of the hip joint, which may cause an effusion. The most common age group is toddlers and early school-age children. The term 'irritable hip' is often used, but in fact this means any hip which is painful when examined, so this is just one cause. The cause is unknown but it may be a reaction to a viral illness. It is a diagnosis of exclusion, so you need to be sure you have considered the other conditions listed above, in particular septic arthritis.

Assessment

The child is most likely to present with a limp but otherwise be perfectly well. This is usually mild (intermittent, slight limp) but can be more severe (non-weight-bearing and marked decrease in range of movement).

Management

See the section 'Distinguishing between transient synovitis and septic arthritis'. Transient synovitis is a benign condition and does not usually recur. It lasts 3–10 days. Since it is a diagnosis of exclusion all cases should be followed up in an appropriate clinic to ensure return to normal within 2 weeks and lack of development of any new symptoms.

Septic arthritis

Assessment

Septic arthritis (bacterial infection within a joint) can develop rapidly over a couple of days. It is usually a result of haematogenous spread from a focus of infection elsewhere, such as throat, ear or skin infection. This sometimes follows secondary infection of vascular access sites or other skin problems, but more often the primary source of the infection is never found. It can affect any large or medium-size joint, e.g. shoulder, knee.

The most common symptom is the child not using the limb, or pain when it is handled (for example, crying because of hip pain when the nappy is changed). Overlying redness or warmth are not common, so you need to keep a high index of suspicion.

Management

See also the section 'Distinguishing between transient synovitis and septic arthritis'. Septic arthritis requires immediate referral for prompt drainage in an operating theatre and IV antibiotic therapy, if long-term complications are to be avoided.

 Children under 3 years are especially vulnerable to septic arthritis!

Distinguishing between septic arthritis and transient synovitis

Transient synovitis is by far the commonest explanation for the 'irritable hip' and can occur at any age, although most frequently between 4–8 years. Septic arthritis can also occur at any age but children under age 3 are especially vulnerable. Distinction between these two potential diagnoses is imperative.

Four findings are considered to be important, and the more that are present the more likely the chance of septic arthritis:

(1) A history of fever
(2) Inability to weight-bear
(3) An erythrocyte sedimentation rate >40 mm/hr
(4) A serum white blood cell count of >12,000 cells/mm^3

Early in the disease process symptoms and signs of the two conditions will be hard to discriminate, and blood markers, especially C-reactive protein, may not have risen. X-rays are normal in both conditions. Ultrasound will identify an effusion in both conditions, confirming that the pathology is within the hip joint.

If there is any suspicion of septic arthritis, the child must be referred to orthopaedics immediately because the joint can be destroyed in a matter of hours, and needs opening and irrigation in an operating theatre. If discharging a child with a limp, advise the parents to return quickly to a hospital if limping worsens or the child develops a fever in the next few days.

Slipped upper femoral epiphysis (SUFE)

This condition is also known as slipped capital femoral epiphysis. It presents with thigh or knee pain. It occurs when the unfused epiphysis of the femoral head slips position. It happens around age 8–15 years (earlier in girls because puberty is earlier). It is more common in boys than girls and both hips can be affected. Two body types are classically, though not necessarily, associated with this condition:

(1) Obese
(2) Tall and thin

The actual slipping of the femoral epiphysis may occur gradually or suddenly, precipitated by minor trauma. There may be a history of a few weeks of more minor symptoms preceding the acute event.

 There may, or may not, be a history of trauma!

Assessment

Remember that the child will commonly complain of thigh or knee pain rather than of hip or groin pain. This is a well-known pitfall but if overlooked will lead to missed or late diagnosis, long-term complications and litigation. The child may be limping or non-weight-bearing. On examination hip movements, particularly internal rotation, may be restricted. Watch the child's face to detect pain, and watch to see if they are tilting their pelvis to compensate.

SUFE may present with isolated thigh or knee pain!

X-ray

You should request a pelvis view to help you to compare with the opposite side, but beware of bilateral disease.

A line drawn along the superior border of the femoral neck (Klein's line) should normally cut through the top of the epiphysis on the AP view. In a slipped upper femoral epiphysis, the whole of the epiphysis may lie below this line (Figure 9.21). On the AP view the earliest signs are widening and irregularity of the physis. Subtle slips will be missed on an AP view; they are better seen on a true lateral. However, to reduce the amount of radiation, a compromise is a 'frog leg' lateral view, where the legs are partly externally rotated (Figure 9.22). If in doubt, seek a radiologist's advice.

Radiological diagnosis can be tricky; further imaging, such as a radioisotope bone scan or CT, may be needed.

Management

If you suspect a slipped upper femoral epiphysis, seek immediate orthopaedic advice. The patient should avoid further weight-bearing.

Perthes avascular necrosis of the femoral head

This is caused by avascular necrosis of the femoral head and presents with hip, thigh or knee pain. It usually affects children in the 5–9 age group, but can happen from 2–16 years. It occurs in boys more frequently than girls, particularly slim, active boys. Anything which affects the vasculature

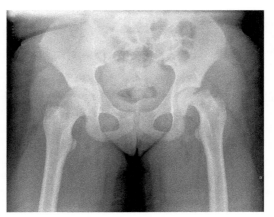

 Figure 9.21 Obvious left slipped upper femoral epiphysis.

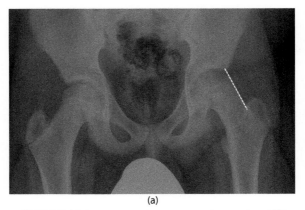

(a)

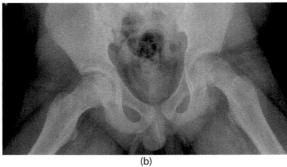

(b)

 Figure 9.22 Subtle left slipped upper femoral epiphysis.

In Figure 9.22a the femoral head lies below Klein's line. In Figure 9.22b the frog leg lateral view enables the slip to be seen more obviously. If in doubt about the diagnosis, seek a radiologist's advice.

of the small vessels which supply the femoral head via the capsule can cause avascular necrosis of the femoral head and give the radiological appearance of Perthes disease; this includes haematological conditions like sickle cell disease, abnormal anatomy or steroid treatment. The term 'Perthes disease' is used when no such explanation for the necrosis can be found, which is more often the case. The condition may be bilateral but rarely affects both hips at the same time. It is unlikely that trauma precipitates Perthes disease, but many parents try to associate limping with recent trauma.

 There may or may not be a history of trauma!

Assessment

Remember that the child will more likely complain of thigh or knee pain than hip or groin pain. The child may be limping or non-weight-bearing. On examination, hip movements, particularly internal rotation, may be limited by pain. Watch the child's face to detect pain, and watch to see if they are tilting their pelvis to compensate.

 Perthes disease may present with isolated thigh or knee pain!

X-ray

X-ray the pelvis to help you to compare with the opposite side. In the initial stages little may be seen on X-ray. Later, the femoral head epiphysis shows patchy sclerosis and fragmentation giving a 'moth-eaten' appearance, and can eventually become flattened (Figure 9.23). If in doubt, seek senior advice. Further imaging, such as magnetic resonance imaging, may be needed for diagnosis.

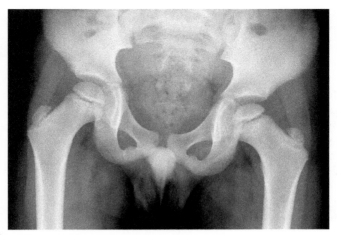

 Figure 9.23 **Left Perthes disease.**

Management

If you diagnose Perthes disease, the condition does not need immediate attention but orthopaedic referral is required.

CHAPTER 10

BURNS, SCALDS AND CHEMICAL AND ELECTRICAL INJURIES

INTRODUCTION

A burn is caused by heat, chemicals, electricity or radiation. A scald is a burn produced by a hot liquid and vapour. This chapter covers all causes except radiation burns. Most minor burns in middle- and high-income countries occur in the home in children 1–3 years old, and are due to hot liquids or contact with household objects, particularly in crowded houses. Burns and scalds may leave permanent scars or abnormal pigmentation. Some of these injuries are preventable, with closer supervision. See Chapter 1, Injury Prevention, and Chapter 14, Non-Accidental Injury. Sunburn can occur due to lack of protection. Actual inflicted burns are much less common and there is a good evidence-based review of this available from the CORE INFO group.

http://www.core-info.cardiff.ac.uk/reviews

If there is not a clear and fluent account of the event, seek senior advice in case of child protection issues!

Major burns are an important cause of death in children worldwide. Some deaths are due to inhalation injury with only minor skin burns. Death is more common in areas of socioeconomic deprivation, and unfortunately neglect and arson are major factors.

HISTORY

Your history needs to take the following factors into account:

- Risk of inhalational injury: possible exposure to smoke or hot gases if in an enclosed space.
- The risk of associated injuries, for example injuries sustained while trying to escape.
- The context of the burn – was there an element of neglect? Was there a delay in presentation or lack of detail in the explanation for the burn, which may imply neglect or non-accidental injury?
- The likely depth of the burn – this depends on the temperature and the duration of contact. Burns from hot fat or oil, or contact with very hot surfaces (e.g. an exhaust pipe) may be full thickness; surfaces with much lower temperature (e.g. a room heating radiator) can also cause full-thickness burns if the duration of contact is long (such as in a post-ictal state).
- A patient at risk of deeper than expected burn, such as patients with poor reflexes (e.g. severe learning difficulties) or poor mobility (physical disability), again because of the duration of contact.
- Factors which will confound your examination e.g. toothpaste put on the burn by the family as a misguided first aid measure.
- Remember that a burn is a wound, so check the tetanus immunisation state of the child (see Chapter 3).

 If there was smoke inhalation, call for senior help.

If there was smoke inhalation, there is a risk of carbon monoxide or cyanide poisoning, and thermal injury to the larynx and bronchi. A full description of this situation is beyond the remit of this book but these complications require time-critical treatments, and senior help is needed.

EXAMINATION

General

Exclude potentially major injuries before concentrating on the burn. Then follow the ABC procedure:

- **A**irway – are there burns, soot or swelling around the mouth and/or nose? Is there stridor?

- **Breathing** – is your patient wheezing or do they have stridor? What are their oxygen saturations?
- **Circulation** – burns do not cause circulatory compromise within a couple of hours, so if signs of shock are present, this should alert you to other injuries.

If you find any of these issues, call for senior help and refer to Advanced Pediatric Life Support or similar guidelines!

After a quick initial ABC assessment, focus on alleviating pain (see Chapter 2) before continuing with your examination. Once this is dealt with, you next need to assess burn depth and size, and check that the child has not become cold (either in the pre-hospital environment or due to cooling first aid measures which have been left on for too long).

Wet dressings left on for too long can cause hypothermia and peripheral shutdown!

Depth of burn

The depth of burn injury is classified in many ways. Americans use the terms first, second and third degree burns. In the UK we use the following classification:

- I – 'Superficial': erythema, which fades in an hour or two
- IIa – 'Superficial dermal': blistered areas with a healthy pink base; this is a partial thickness burn
- IIb – 'Deep dermal': blistered areas with a mottled, pale base; this is also a partial thickness burn
- III – 'Full thickness': the burn appears white, brown or charred, and lacks sensation

In practice, burn depth is difficult to assess in the acute situation and many burns are of mixed depth; if you are unsure seek advice. After 24–48 hours it is usually much easier to estimate burn severity.

Size of burn

The area of skin which has been injured is expressed as a percentage of the body surface area (BSA). Areas of simple erythema (red skin without blistering) are not included in the BSA calculation but are a common

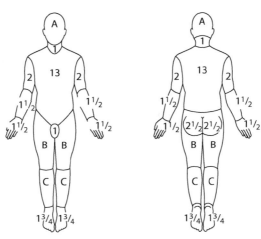

Percentage of body surface area

Area	Age 1	5	10
A=$1/_2$ of head	$9^1/_2$ $8^1/_2$	$6^1/_2$	$5^1/_2$
B=$1/_2$ of one thigh	$2^3/_4$ $3^1/_4$	4	$4^1/_2$
C=$1/_2$ of one leg	$2^1/_2$ $2^1/_2$	$2^3/_4$	3

 Figure 10.1 Lund and Browder charts for assessment of burn area in children.

cause of over-estimation of the size of the burn. For small areas of burn the simplest method is to calculate 1% as the area of the child's hand (including the fingers, not just the palm). A burns chart can help you calculate the BSA (Figure 10.1). The burns chart for children under 5 years is different from older children and adults because of their different head and body proportions. The chart also allows you to draw the burn, which makes your notes easier to understand.

Pattern of the burn

If the burn involves important areas like the eyes, genitalia or nipples, this will require specialist involvement. Check that the pattern of burn matches the history exactly, to be sure of no child protection issues. Scalds cause a splash pattern, contact burns should match the shape of the object contacted.

MANAGEMENT

First aid treatment

If the burn has not already been cooled, run cold water over the burn for 5 minutes or immerse the limb in cold water. Then gently dry and protect the burn from air movement, which causes pain. Often cling wrap (as used for food) is the quickest solution. A non-adhesive dressing takes longer to do and more members of staff may want to see the injury before definitive dressing.

 Do not leave wet cloths on the burned areas as this can cause hypothermia!

Initially creams or ointments should not be put on the burned areas. Parents may apply these or other inappropriate substances such as toothpaste or butter to the burn. This should be gently discouraged for potential future accidents, and the correct first aid advice given.

Medical treatment

 Treat pain before making a detailed assessment of the burn itself!

Pain is always present in minor burn injury because nerve endings in the skin have been damaged and are exposed. Therefore covering the burn is the best way of soothing pain. Calm the carer and the child and use distraction if necessary. Intranasal opiate can be useful in calming the child (and therefore everyone else) down (see Chapter 2). Supplement this with oral analgesia and keep the burn covered until the analgesia is working.

For definitive burn dressing the wounds should gently be cleaned with water first. Initially the wounds should be dressed with a non-stick dressing such as paraffin gauze. More expensive silver-based dressings can be used. Some dressings distort the appearance of the burn when reviewed at follow-up so only use these if the person likely to review the burn is experienced in burn management. To apply effective dressings see Chapter 15. Facial wounds are very difficult to dress so can be left exposed and a petroleum-based ointment applied regularly.

Referral and follow-up

Burns which should be referred for same-day specialist advice are those involving more than 10% BSA, any with full thickness areas and those in special areas, e.g. around the eyes, mouth, perineum or nappy area or nipple. For the remainder, the location of follow-up will depend on local guidelines, ranging from burn clinics run by plastic surgeons, to emergency department clinics, through to nurse-led clinics at the family doctor's practice.

As we mentioned in the previous section, non-stick dressings such as paraffin gauze are best for the early days when serous fluid will still ooze out. Subsequently, drier non-stick dressings such as silicon-based dressings are useful. After the first day or two dressing changes should be minimised and left for 4–5 days if not dirty, to avoid disturbing healing tissues.

Advice for parents is important at this stage. They should be told to look out for the signs of toxic shock syndrome (see the next section) over the next 5 days. They should be advised to give analgesia before leaving home for the planned dressing change. As the burn heals, it will probably go through an itchy phase, and emollient creams used for eczema can help the itch. The affected skin should be protected from sunshine for the next 12 months, as it will burn easily. Finally, the parents should not worry about the colour of the scar until the second year after injury, as it is usually more obvious in the first year.

COMPLICATIONS

Localised infection

This is rare in the first 48 hours. Erythema around burns is common, and does not need to be treated with systemic antibiotics. Infection can be difficult to diagnose and prevents wound healing. You should suspect infection if the burn is painful, the erythema is spreading, the wound has an offensive smell, there is excessive oozing or if the child is systemically unwell (see 'Toxic shock syndrome'). Mild local infection may clear with daily dressings. If you choose to prescribe antibiotics, ensure a wound review within 48 hours. Infection should be treated with an anti-streptococcal and anti-staphylococcal oral antibiotic such as flucloxacillin or erythroycin. Swabs for microbiological culture should be taken.

Toxic shock syndrome

This is much more common in children than adults and can occur in a child with a very minor burn. It is caused by toxin-secreting bacteria, either streptococcus or staphylococcus, although the burn itself often does not look infected. It usually presents at 2–5 days after the burn. Prognosis is related to time to diagnosis, with delay leading to death in some cases. The presenting symptoms are fever, rash and watery diarrhoea. Clinically the child may be shocked and may progress to need intensive care quite rapidly.

Take suspected toxic shock syndrome seriously! Give anti-staphylococcal IV antibiotics as soon as suspected, consider IV fluids and involve senior help and the intensive care team early.

CHEMICAL INJURIES

General information

Chemical injuries most commonly occur due to cleaning agents in the house. Most cleaning fluids are gentle but beware the extra-powerful or industrial-use varieties. Check the pH of the affected area, then rinse with running water until further facts are established. For chemical injuries to the eyes, see Chapter 4. Specific antidotes are rarely necessary but advice should be sought. In the UK there is the National Poisons Information Service; the website is called Toxbase. If the chemical has been brought in by the family, it is useful to test it using litmus paper to see if it is acid or alkaline.

 http://www.toxbase.org

Acids

Acid substances usually cause immediate pain, but most burns are superficial because acids cause coagulation of the surface tissues, forming a protective barrier to further damage. Treat by irrigation using 500 ml of saline, using an IV administration set. Repeat if pain is still present.

Alkalis

Alkalis are found in household cleaning products, and may be highly concentrated in substances such as oven cleaner or drain unblocker. For ingested alkalis, see Chapter 12. Alkalis permeate between cell membranes, causing deep-seated damage. Deceptively, they may be less painful than acids initially.

 Alkaline injuries are more serious than acid injuries!

Treat in the same way initially as acids, by irrigation; however, it may take several hours and many litres of irrigation for the burn to become pain-free. Litmus paper is not useful for monitoring response to irrigation. It is just used to see if the injury is acid or alkaline. Response to treatment is judged by symptoms. The subsequent management of any chemical burn is the same as a thermal burn (just discussed).

ELECTRICAL INJURIES

Electrical injuries may cause cardiac dysrhythmias, deep burns and deep soft tissue damage.

History

Was this a domestic voltage supply or a potential high-voltage injury? Young children sustain electrical burns in the home when they poke metal objects into live sockets or they touch live wires. This type of electrical injury is low voltage. Much more serious injuries occur with high-voltage supplies like a telegraph wire or an electricity substation or railway track. In any electrical accident check for a cardiac dysrhythmia in the history if the child is old enough to describe feeling faint or having palpitations.

Patients who have injuries due to high-voltage electricity may have severe injuries in addition to a major burn!

Examination

Check the child's pulse. If it is fast or irregular perform a 12-lead ECG and a rhythm strip. If the child is in sinus rhythm and has no ectopic beats when first monitored there is no need for further monitoring. Look at where the skin touched the electricity supply to examine the 'entry point'. Assess in the same way as a non-electrical burn (discussed previously). Next look for an 'exit point' – this is where the current can leave the skin as it exits the body – e.g. a finger on the opposite hand or through a foot.

These two things will give you a picture of the trajectory of the current and therefore tell you where to look for underlying damage. Often there is no exit point, so rely on symptoms to see where the affected areas may be. Damage to deeper structures between entry and exit points can result in compartment syndrome developing (see Chapter 3). Make sure you palpate the muscles for tenderness and test movement of the muscles for pain.

Ask for senior advice if you suspect a dysrhythmia or high-voltage injury!

Lightning can kill, but survivors are more common. Dysrhythmias and respiratory or cardiac arrest may occur on scene. The skin may have a pathognomonic fern- or feather-like pattern, and deep-seated soft tissue injury is common.

Management

Seek senior advice for high-voltage injuries. Otherwise, if there is no evidence of dysrhythmia or compartment syndrome you can discharge the child but give the parents advice about the symptoms and signs of compartment syndrome (see Chapter 3).

HEAT ILLNESS AND HYPOTHERMIA

Heat illness

In prolonged exposure to heat from external sources or prolonged exercise, children may develop:

- Heat cramps
- Heat exhaustion – irritability, dizziness, headache, nausea
- Heat stroke – temperature over 41°C, shock, coma, convulsions

These may be associated with sunburn. The cause is fluid loss from sweating, with inadequate replacement of water and salt. Children with cystic fibrosis are at greater risk.

Standard oral rehydration solutions are usually adequate in the early stages. In heat exhaustion and heat stroke intravenous replacement is needed. When the core temperature is over 39.5°C clothes should be removed and the child should be sponged with tepid water. A fan of cold air can be used with caution – if the skin is cooled too rapidly then capillary vasoconstriction occurs and the core temperature rises further.

This is a rare and serious condition! Seek senior help.

Hypothermia

Children have larger body surface areas than adults, so can lose heat easily. After accidents outdoors, particularly in wet or icy weather, hypothermia can occur. Drowning accidents are beyond the scope of this book. Mild hypothermia (above 33°C) will respond to warm blankets, warming mattresses (such as the chemically activated Transwarmer®) and warmed drinks or warmed IV fluids. At 32°C or below more aggressive measures are needed, which are outside the scope of this book.

CHAPTER 11

BITES, STINGS AND ALLERGIC REACTIONS

BITES IN GENERAL

History

Bites from various animals are quite common in children. Regardless of the source of the bite, for the most part the general principles of wound management apply (see Chapter 3), including checking the child's tetanus vaccination status. Bites are usually heavily contaminated with bacteria, and the wound edges are often irregular or crushed. Depending on the size of the animal, there may be quite a significant crush component, including the possibility of an underlying fracture (e.g. from a large dog).

Examination

Assess the wound for the extent of crush injury, the state of the wound edges, damage to deep structures such as nerves, vessels, tendons and bones and any possibility of joint penetration. Consider whether this is a puncture wound or a small open wound, or whether cleaning and repair under general anaesthesia may be needed, for example either a large wound or one with the potential for joint capsule penetration.

Management

Manage all bites as contaminated wounds (see Chapter 3), and do not be falsely reassured by small wounds. Consider X-rays if you suspect a fracture or foreign body (e.g. a broken tooth if bitten by an older dog).

 The risk of infection is increased in puncture versus open wounds!

Explore and irrigate the wound thoroughly (see Chapter 15). Avoid closure with sutures if possible – you can draw the wound edges a little closer together to aid healing but avoid closing the skin, so that infection can easily drain from the wound. If the cosmetic effect of allowing healing by secondary intention is too great, get advice from a plastic or orofacialmaxillary surgeon.

It is not strictly necessary, but is common practice to treat animal bites with broad-spectrum antibiotics such as coamoxyclavulanic acid. For advice on tetanus immunoglobulin, see Chapter 3. Consider rabies prophylaxis if the child was bitten in an area where rabies is present.

HUMAN BITES

History

The human mouth carries large numbers of aerobic and anaerobic bacteria, which means that bites have a high risk of infection. If the person who bit the patient is known to have, or is at risk of, hepatitis or HIV infection, consider whether there may be transmission of the virus. Follow your local guidelines if you think the child is at risk.

Remember the history of a bite may not be clear, for example a wound from a punch-type injury or in child maltreatment!

Examination and Management

See bites in general. For management, prophylactic antibiotics are required to cover both aerobic and anaerobic bacteria, e.g. coamoxyclavulanic acid. Consider hepatitis B and/or HIV prophylaxis, depending on your local guidelines.

DOG BITES

History

The child may have been very frightened by the event. The size of dog is important, as a bite from a large dog is associated with significant soft tissue and bone injury. Ask about the circumstances of the bite to ensure there was no irresponsible behaviour or neglect, or if the dog may pose a risk to others, in which case you may have to contact the police if the family has not already done so. In the UK some breeds of dog are covered by the Dangerous Dogs Act. If the dog is known by the family to be potentially aggressive, child protection procedures may need to be followed.

Consider whether there were issues of child safety in the incident, and whether the animal still poses a threat to others!

Examination and Management

See bites in general.

CAT BITES

History and examination are the same as bites in general. The most common organism to cause infection is *Pasteurella multocida*, which is found as a commensal in the mouths of cats. This can lead to severe wound sepsis with associated septicaemia. Coamoxyclavulanic acid is a suitable antibiotic for management.

SNAKE BITES

History

Try to identify the snake. The only poisonous snake native to the UK is the adder (*Vipera berus*). Adder bites generally only lead to local symptoms. More serious bites from imported snakes (envenomation) are occasionally seen. Systemic symptoms include respiratory distress, vomiting, abdominal pain or diarrhoea.

Examination

Local effects include pain, swelling, bruising and enlargement of regional lymph nodes. Systemic signs of envenoming are hypotension, angioedema, depressed level of consciousness, ECG abnormalities, spontaneous bleeding, coagulopathy, respiratory distress and acute renal failure.

Management

If the bite is on a limb, the whole limb should be bandaged with a compression bandage and immobilised to reduce systemic effects. Do not apply a tourniquet. For specific treatments, follow local guidelines or use a toxicology reference source such as (in the UK) the National Poisons Information Service.

 http://www.toxbase.org

If there are any signs of envenomation, assess and treat ABC, before focussing on specific treatments!

INSECT BITES

Insect bites may occur without a clear history. Symptoms within the first 48 hours are caused by a localised allergic response causing itching, erythema and swelling. After this time, erythema and swelling may indicate secondary bacterial infection.

Management

Keep the area cool, and consider topical or oral antihistamines. If secondary bacterial infection is suspected (after 48 hours) then give oral antibiotic, e.g. flucloxacillin.

STINGS

Bee and wasp stings

Bee and wasp stings usually present as localised pain and swelling. Treat as for insect bites. Rarely a sting may lead to a generalised severe anaphylactic response in a susceptible individual. If the stinger is still present (e.g. from a bee) remove it. Examine for any effect on airway, breathing, circulation, gastrointestinal tract and skin. For skin and gastrointestinal tract, treatment with oral antihistamine is enough. For more severe symptoms, administer intramuscular adrenaline quickly. Further discussion of anaphylaxis is outside the scope of this book.

Jellyfish stings

Stings from jellyfish in the waters around the UK lead to local irritation only. Treat as for insect bites. Other countries tend to have local guidelines.

FOREIGN BODIES

SOFT TISSUES

Presentation to the emergency department with a foreign body (FB) is very common. Your management will depend upon:

- The site
- The size
- The presence or absence of infection
- The length of time the FB has been there
- The nature of the FB

 It is important to do no further harm when trying to remove an FB!

Some FBs are better left in situ, until or unless they are causing a problem. The next sections will help you balance this judgement call.

Nature of the FB

Organic FBs are more likely to cause infections and other complications, whereas some inorganic FBs such as small pieces of glass or air gun pellets can remain in situ for life, or at least many years, before causing problems.

Site

Think before you try to remove an FB. For instance, are you in dangerous territory, such as near blood vessels or important nerves? Might you have to extend the wound to get it out? If so, could you be running into joints, nerves or tendons? If there is a risk of this, you need a surgeon to remove the FB. A good knowledge of anatomy and a clear view are needed.

If in doubt, refer to a surgeon!

Size

If the FB requires a large anaesthetic field for its removal, calculate the maximum safe dose of anaesthetic you may use for the size of the child. If you are likely to exceed this dose, refer for general anaesthesia. If the FB itself is large, do not underestimate where it could be penetrating. FBs can be like icebergs: innocent-looking, but much larger below the surface.

Infection

If infection is present (cellulitis or abscess), the FB needs to be removed, regardless of its nature or site.

Duration

If the wound has closed (24–48 hours), even an FB which looks superficial on X-ray may be very difficult to remove. Unless it is easily palpable under the skin, refer to a surgeon.

Splinters

These are commonly found in hands or under nails. Splinters should be removed using 'splinter forceps'. These are a special kind of forceps with a very fine point – always use them as they make removal much easier. Small pieces of splinter or dirt remaining far under the nail after the main splinter has been removed should be left alone – most wood softens to a pulp in a few days and will come out with a bead of pus. If splinters in the skin are small and break off, leave them for a few days. They generally work their own way out.

Fish hooks

These are usually embedded in fingers. There are two methods of removal, depending on the size of the barb. Small barbs may simply be pulled out, although an incision may be necessary to enlarge the wound. Larger barbs may have to be 'pushed through'. The shaft is fed in to the finger until the barb starts to cause bulging of the overlying skin. A scalpel is then used to create an exit point for the barb, then the whole thing is fed through this new incision.

Glass

Glass can be very difficult to spot in a wound. Most glass is radio-opaque. If the glass broke into multiple shards, an occult FB is possible, so an X-ray is needed. Once the FB has been removed, a confirmatory X-ray is needed (Figure 12.1).

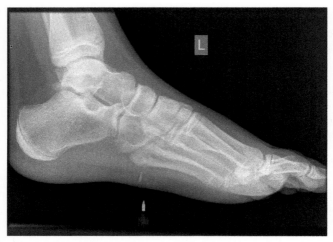

 Figure 12.1 Glass FB in foot.

 Have a low threshold for requesting a soft tissue X-ray for wounds caused by glass!

Role of ultrasound

Soft tissue ultrasound is a good method of identifying the presence of an FB, although the accuracy of ultrasound depends on the level of operator experience.

THE EYE

See Chapter 4 for general information and Chapter 15 for removal of foreign bodies.

THE EAR

External Auditory Canal

Assessment

Insertion of an FB into the ear is very common in young children. Usually the child confesses, either on the day or sometimes days or weeks later. In others there is no clear history of an FB, and the child presents with pain or discharge from the ear. Occasionally live insects can enter the ear. An FB such as a bead in the ear canal can be quite painful, and to permit examination or removal the child may need strong analgesia, for example intranasal opiate, which is useful for both analgesia and anxiolysis (see Chapter 2).

The FB is usually clearly seen with an auriscope. Sometimes the discharge is too thick to allow the FB to be seen. Such cases are usually diagnosed after referral to an ear, nose and throat (ENT or otolaryngology) clinic.

Management
See Chapter 15. Two percent lidocaine solution can assist with removal as well as helping with pain.

EMBEDDED EARRINGS

Assessment
Stud type earrings can become embedded within the pinna. Most commonly the back or 'butterfly' becomes embedded, with inflammation and sometimes infection. If swelling is severe the front of the earring may also become embedded.

Management
The earring is usually easily removed with an inferior auricular nerve block, which is invaluable (see Chapter 15). Once pain-free, apply gentle pressure to the front of the earring to release the butterfly at the back. Occasionally a small skin incision over the butterfly is required. Remove the whole earring. If the pinna is infected antibiotics may be required, although simply removing the earring is often sufficient.

THE NOSE

Assessment

FB insertion into the nose is also very common in young children. Usually the child confesses, either on the day or sometimes days or weeks later. In others there is no clear history of an FB, and the child presents with pain or discharge from the nose. Lie the child back with their head extended and use the light of an auriscope to look up the nostril. The FB is usually obvious.

Management

Before resorting to pinning the child down and using instruments to extract the FB, try the much more child-friendly 'kissing' technique (see Chapter 15).

HAIR TOURNIQUET SYNDROME

Assessment

This odd condition occurs when one or more hairs become wrapped around the base of a digit, and gradually constrict, causing ischaemia. It usually occurs in babies, and affects fingers and toes, but may affect other areas such as the penis. It is most common in toddlers and babies. There is no history of a hair becoming entangled – you will only make the diagnosis by being aware of this condition or by very close examination. The digit may be bluish or white. A magnifying glass may be needed to see the hair(s).

Management

The hair must be released as soon as possible. Hair dissolving creams, such as those commercially available cosmetically for adults, are useful. Apply the cream, cover with a non-porous dressing and leave for no more than 15 minutes. Remove and rinse. Do not do this if the skin has already broken down.

If this does not work, cut or unwind the hair using forceps; a stitch cutter may be able to get under the hair. The hair may be wrapped several times around the digit, so it is possible to only partially relieve the ischaemia. Keep the child under observation for an hour until you are sure. If you are unsure that you have successfully released the hair, call for a more experienced person. The child may end up needing general anaesthesia, a hand surgeon and an operating microscope. A deep incision may have to be made.

Be sure the digit looks healthy and reperfused before discharging the child!

SWALLOWED FOREIGN BODIES

The throat

Assessment

Usually the child will have ingested something sharp, such as a bone, and have felt it get 'stuck'. Another common situation is if a child has tried to swallow a coin. The majority of children are able to describe their symptoms. Quite often, the FB has descended into the stomach and it is the abrasion which is still felt.

If there is any history of choking consider inhalation (see 'Upper airway' section)!

If the child is distressed, call for senior help! Do not upset the child further, or send them for an X-ray.

If the child is cooperative, examine the throat (see Chapter 15) and if the FB cannot be seen, it may be behind the fauces, on the tonsil. If the child will cooperate, spray the throat with lidocaine anaesthetic, use a tongue depressor spatula to push the anterior fauces to one side, and the bone may come into view.

Imaging
If examination of the mouth does not reveal an FB, consider whether it is radio-opaque, and will therefore be seen on a soft tissue lateral neck X-ray.

Fish bones may or may not show up, depending on the size and type of bone; ask your radiographer for advice.

Management
If the FB is visualised, remove it with forceps if the child is cooperative. You may need lidocaine spray to achieve this. If the FB is visible in the hypopharynx or oesophagus on X-ray, refer to the ENT specialists. If the FB has not shown up on X-ray or is not radio-opaque, your management depends on the degree of distress. If the child is distressed, refer to the ENT specialists. However, the majority of children can go home with simple analgesia, be encouraged to drink and eat soft foods and attend an outpatient clinic 24 hours later if symptoms persist – symptoms of a scratch will be improving at this stage.

The oesophagus
The commonest object to get stuck in the oesophagus is a coin. Other FBs can be managed similarly. Two less common but more dangerous situations are swallowed magnets and swallowed button batteries (see 'Button battery ingestion and insertion') which can be life-threatening and require a different approach.

Old-fashioned (ferrite) magnets are largely innocuous unless two are swallowed, and stick together in the gastrointestinal tract. More recently, children can swallow multiple neodymium magnets, which are increasingly used in toys. These will stick together and can cause bowel perforation and bleeding. It is probably safest to follow the same management as for button batteries (see the next section).

Coins usually pass through the oesophagus with no problem, but can become stuck. Common places for the FB to lodge are at the crico-pharyngeus level or the oesophago-gastric junction, although some can become stuck in the middle third of the oesophagus.

Assessment

The child may give a history of ingestion or be witnessed swallowing an FB. The parent or carer may give a history of items last seen with the child that are now missing or alternatively the child may be found retching or choking. Coughing is a good clue that the FB may actually be in the airway (see 'Inhaled foreign bodies'). Sitting forward and drooling usually suggests an FB at the level of the crico-pharyngeus muscle in the neck. Children with middle or lower third FBs (gastro-oesophageal junction) usually complain of retro-sternal pain.

In a child with a 'swallowed' FB, check the history specifically for coughing!

Imaging

X-rays may be useful (if the situation is stable). Swallowed coins in asymptomatic children who are able to communicate well (aged 4 and above) do not require imaging. A lateral neck X-ray can help confirm that the FB is behind the airway, i.e. in the oesophagus (Figure 12.2). Request a neck to upper abdomen X-ray, which will avoid irradiating the gonads. You only need to know that there is not an FB proximal to the pylorus.

Management

Foreign bodies in the mouth and upper throat were discussed previously. Once an FB reaches the stomach, most will pass through the gastrointestinal tract uneventfully. Figure 12.3 provides an algorithm for a swallowed FB. If discharging the child, advise the parents that complications are very unlikely, but that they should return if the child starts vomiting, refusing to eat or complaining of abdominal pain. Searching the child's stools can be discouraged!

Button battery ingestion and insertion

This is an increasing problem with the widespread use of electronic equipment and toys in households. They emit an electric field which causes

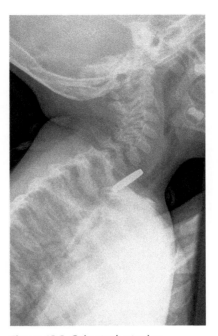

 Figure 12.2 Coin stuck at crico-pharyngeus muscle in oesophagus, clearly visible behind airway.

lysis of surrounding tissues, and can cause life-threatening injuries within 2 hours of ingestion, such as aorto-enteric fistula. In areas like the ear and nose, severe erosion of surrounding tissues can occur. Serious complications are more likely with the larger (20 mm and 25 mm) batteries. Deaths have been reported from 2 hours post-ingestion up to a month afterwards.

 Beware button batteries – they can kill within hours!

Any child presenting with significant haematemesis should be suspected of swallowing a button battery (Figure 12.4), even if there has been no suggestion of this happening, unless the child has another clear cause for haematemesis (i.e. a significant past medical history). As soon as the possibility of button battery ingestion is raised, follow the guidance in Figure 12.5 as fast as possible, and get senior help.

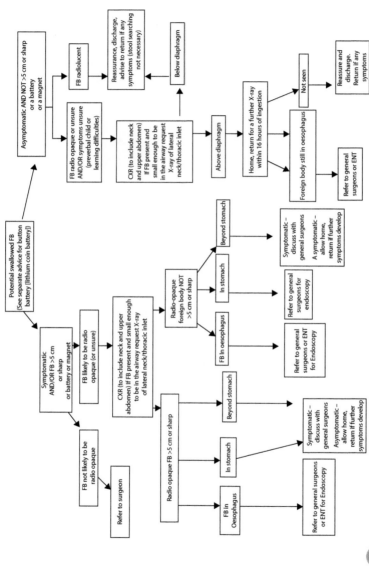

Figure 12.3 Management of a swallowed FB.

Button (lithium coin) battery ingestion or insertion

Symptomatic
Haematemesis
Airway obstruction or drooling.
Dysphagia or acute refusal to eat.
Choking or acute difficulty breathing.

Asymptomatic
No respiratory concerns, eating
and drinking ok. No haematemesis.

Assess **ABC. Prepare for
resuscitation.
alert senior doctors.**
Contact anaesthetist and
surgeon.
Arrange for immediate neck
to upper abdomen X-Ray.

Keep nil by mouth.
Arrange for immediate neck to
upper abdomen X-Ray (if ingestion)
or X-Ray of appropriate part
(if insertion).

In oesophagus

Button battery present
Keep child calm! Insert 2 large IV/IO
lines. Urgent blood cross-match
10 ml/kg. Alert operating theatres
and consider Tranexamic acid (TXA).

BB in
oesophagus

Co-ordinate
with surgical
team to
remove via
very urgent
endoscopy.

Below diaphragm in stomach
Repeat an X-Ray in 8–12 hours
after time of ingestion.
If still present seek surgical advice.

Beyond stomach
These generally all pass without
incident and parents do not need
to check stool. Must return if any
symptoms.

Key points
Ingestion of button batteries can kill even if the child presents asymptomatically.
There may be no history of swallowing a battery at all so suspect BB in any child
with significant haematemesis and no known cause.

Figure 12.4 Management of a swallowed button battery (lithium/coin battery).

 Consider the possibility of button battery ingestion for any child presenting with a significant haematemesis!

 Get senior and specialist help immediately if a button battery is in the oropharynx or oesophagus!

Detergent capsules

In recent years there has been a growing awareness of the dangers of capsules and tablets used in dishwashers, and in washing machines in particular. These look very attractive to children, as they look like sweets. They contain strong

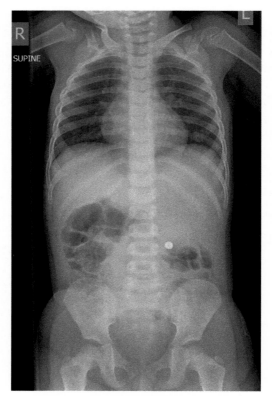

 Figure 12.5 Button battery through the pylorus and into the intestines.

alkaline compounds which can cause quite severe erosion of the oropharynx and oesophagus when swallowed. They should be managed by encouraging drinking several glasses of water within the first couple of hours post-ingestion. The child should be kept under observation for 8 hours and a specialist (usually ENT) involved if they become symptomatic from the throat or oesophagus. Side effects also include drowsiness – if this happens, seek advice from your country's toxicology service.

 http://www.toxbase.org in the UK

INHALED FOREIGN BODIES

Inhaled foreign bodies occur most commonly in pre-school-age children. Almost anything can be inhaled; foods such as peanuts and sweets, and beads are the commonest culprits. Sadly, inhaled FBs causing severe airway obstruction can result in death at home or en route to hospital.

The history of inhaled FB is usually, but not always, clear. Always suspect an FB if there is a sudden onset of choking or stridor. Sometimes an FB may present several weeks or months later, and can be mistaken for asthma or a recurrent chest infection.

Upper airway

Children with complete airway obstruction rarely survive to hospital. In those who reach hospital there is most likely to be stridor, gagging, choking or drooling. Sometimes the child may just be very quiet and apprehensive and sitting with an upright posture, in which they are most comfortable. If this is the case it is imperative not to upset the child further. Crying and struggling may convert a partially obstructed airway into a completely obstructed one.

 Proceed to a resuscitation area but keep the child as calm as possible! Call for senior help.

Encourage and reassure the child whilst awaiting senior help. Use the time to prepare equipment such as Magill forceps and equipment for intubation and needle cricothyroidotomy, and call an operating department technician to help prepare you. Sevoflurane for gaseous induction can be useful.

The method you use depends on symptoms and the age of the child. Back blows can be used in all age groups (Figure 12.6). The Heimlich manoeuvre can be used in children aged 4 and above (Figure 12.7). In younger children there is a risk of injury to abdominal organs so chest thrusts are recommended instead (Figure 12.8).

Lower airway

Assessment

If an FB passes through the main bronchus to the lower airways, a child will present with persistent cough or wheeze or recurrent chest infection. This may be hours to months after the event. On examination there may localised

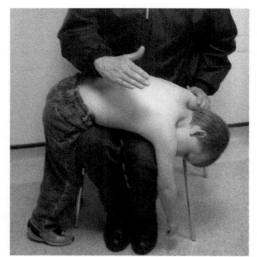

Figure 12.6 Back blows.

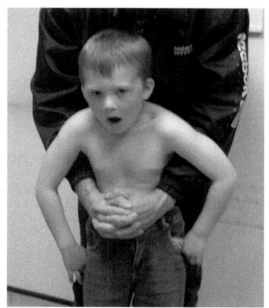

Figure 12.7 The Heimlich manoeuvre.

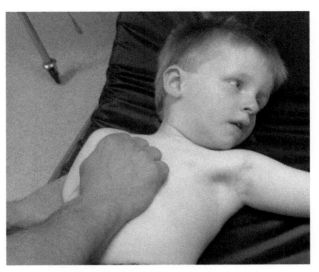

 Figure 12.8 **Chest thrusts in infants.**

wheezing or absent breath sounds. However, examination may be normal. Children can present with signs of wheezing, a pneumonia or empyema with no clue to an inhaled FB. The FB is often discovered at bronchoscopy.

 Beware delayed presentation of FBs in the lower airway!

Imaging
A chest X-ray should be performed for an acute inhalation of an FB, or in the chronic situation, for atypical wheezing or recurrent chest infections. The FB is often not radio-opaque. In 90% of acute cases there is hyperinflation of the lung distal to the FB which can act as a ball-valve, allowing air to enter but not be expelled from the obstructed segment. This is best seen in an expiratory film. In Figure 12.9 you can also see tracheal shift to the right. In the remainder of cases (particularly with a delay in presentation or diagnosis) there are signs of collapse of the obstructed segment of lung (Figure 12.10).

Management
Refer for removal of FB by bronchoscopy under general anaesthesia.

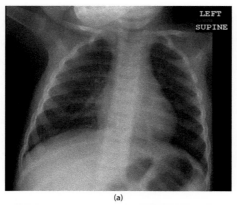

(a)

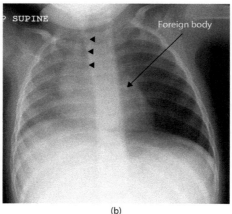

Foreign body

(b)

Figure 12.9 Chest X-Ray in (a) inspiration and (b) expiration demonstrating hyperinflation of left lung (due to 'ball valve' effect). The arrowheads demonstrate tracheal shift to the right.

The inspiratory film was virtually normal. In a child who is too young to cooperate with expiratory views lateral decubitus views may be used. Discuss this with your radiographer.

VAGINAL AND RECTAL FOREIGN BODIES

Assessment

A vaginal or rectal FB is unusual in children. Although simple experimentation occurs, consider if there is any inappropriate sexualised

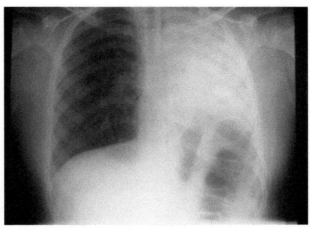

 Figure 12.10 **Left lung collapse a few days after inhaled FB.**

behaviour (suggestive of sexual abuse or exposure to pornography). The child may confess and present acutely, or may present later with discharge or pain. Adolescent girls may present with a history of a lost tampon, or a lost condom.

 Stop to consider sexual abuse or inappropriate exposure and seek senior advice if you are concerned!

Management

All young children with suspected vaginal or rectal FB should be referred for further specialist assessment. It is not appropriate to perform a vaginal or rectal examination of a young child in the emergency department. In adolescents, removal of a lost tampon or other vaginal FB is often simple. If the FB is a lost condom or other sexual item, remember to consider the maturity of the girl, the appropriateness or consensuality of the sexual liaison and issues such as post-coital contraception and sexually transmitted diseases (refer if necessary to Chapters 14, Non-accidental injury, if you have some concerns). Seek senior help if you are unsure.

CHAPTER 13

INJURIES OF THE EXTERNAL GENITALIA AND ANUS

INTRODUCTION

Injury to the genital area usually happens as a result of straddle injuries in girls (e.g. across a bathtub side or bicycle cross-bar) and zip injuries in boys. Other injuries are uncommon. Staff may feel insecure in dealing with injuries in this area, as non-accidental injury has got to be borne in mind. As always, non-accidental injury will be picked up by spotting a history which is flawed, lacks detail or lacks plausibility, in combination with an injury pattern which is either not typical of the mechanism stated, or is unusual (see Chapter 14). In fact, in the UK 99% of these injuries presenting to an emergency department are pure accidents, and those which are not include self-harm as well as sexual abuse. Non-traumatic vaginal discharge and vaginal or rectal bleeding are not covered in this book.

There is obviously a degree of psychological distress associated with injuries in this area. Many children presenting to the emergency department have bled immediately after the incident. This alarms parents but fortunately most have stopped bleeding by the time they reach hospital. Injuries in this area are painful, as the genital area has a rich nerve supply. This can lead to urinary retention. Some children have discomfort on passing urine at presentation and blood in the urine may be described. This is rarely from the urethra, usually being contamination by blood from the injured genitalia.

From about 4 years old, children can be embarrassed or anxious about examination of the area. It is important to look calm, be reassuring and to examine children in privacy. It is wise to involve a chaperone (as experienced as possible), and to avoid repeated examination of the child by getting the right colleague for a second opinion if you need one.

FEMALE GENITAL INJURIES

History

Blunt injury

A fall onto a hard object, particularly a straddle-type injury such as astride the bath or gymnasium or play equipment, is the commonest cause of injury to female external genitalia. The direct force involved leads to compression of the soft tissues of the vulva between the object and the pelvis. A punch or kick to the genital area gives similar findings to a fall onto a hard object. This assault may be unintentional in rough play.

Stretch injury

When females accidentally do 'the splits' this can result in superficial lacerations of the skin of the perineum or posterior fourchette, especially if labial adhesions are present.

Accidental penetrating injury

This mechanism is less common but potentially more damaging than the others. Take a careful history and stop to consider whether the story may be untrue. Listen to the detail and use accessory sources of information (see Chapter 14).

Examination

Blunt injury causes bruising, abrasions and/or lacerations, which are usually anterior and asymmetrical. Lacerations tend to be superficial and are most commonly found between the labia majora and labia minora. Bruising of the soft tissues may be severe but the hymen is not damaged. For penetrating injuries, make sure that the full depth of penetration can be visualised. If superficial, manage as above. If not, refer to an experienced surgeon.

 Some penetrating injuries are deceptively deep and require surgical exploration and repair!

When examining the female genitalia, be precise when describing the injured areas. Figure 13.1 can help you with terminology and anatomy. Some EDs use a customised body stamp to improve documentation. Most accidental injuries involve the anterior area or the sides, and are fairly superficial. Be more suspicious about posterior injuries involving the vaginal orifice or deeper injuries, particularly involving the hymen.

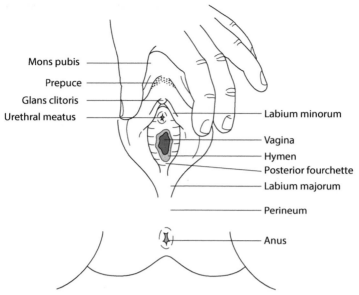

Mons pubis

Prepuce

Glans clitoris

Urethral meatus

Labium minorum

Vagina

Hymen

Posterior fourchette

Labium majorum

Perineum

Anus

Figure 13.1 The female perineum.

If in doubt, seek a second opinion from a more experienced colleague!

Management

Clean all abrasions and superficial lacerations gently with normal saline. Advise frequent warm baths or very gentle showering of the affected area, avoiding soap. Most will heal within a week. Advise the parents to give frequent analgesia and plenty of oral fluids so that weak urine is passed frequently, so as to avoid urinary retention. If urinary retention occurs, this can be managed by maximising analgesia and giving lots of encouragement to pass urine. Sometimes the child can be put in a warm bath and encouraged to let the urine go, into the bath.

MALE EXTERNAL GENITAL INJURIES

Zip injury

The foreskin or shaft of the penis may get caught in a zipper, causing an abrasion or superficial laceration. The zip can be disengaged by cutting its distal end off and separating the two halves. A penile block may be needed and is relatively straightforward – ask for senior advice. A sedative analgesic such as intranasal opiate, or procedural sedation/general anaesthesia, may be necessary (see Chapter 2).

Penile blunt injury

Most penile injuries in childhood are due to a fall onto a hard surface (straddle injury) or an object falling onto the penis. These result in contusions and superficial lacerations. Clean all abrasions and superficial lacerations thoroughly with normal saline. Advise frequent baths or very gentle showering of the affected area, avoiding soap. Most will heal within a week. Advise the parents to give frequent analgesia and plenty of oral fluids so that weak urine is passed frequently, so as to avoid urinary retention.

 Beware of a large haematoma following minor trauma – this could be a ruptured corpus cavernosus which needs surgical exploration!

Penile strangulation injury

The base of the penis can become strangulated either by accident (see hair tourniquet syndrome, Chapter 12) or deliberately, by the child putting something around the penis. The object acts as a tourniquet and the penis becomes swollen distal to the tight band. Urgent release of the constriction is necessary in order to restore the circulation. Try to remove the constricting object, but when the area is very swollen or the object is metal, expert help and general anaesthesia with removal in the operating theatre may be needed.

Injuries to the scrotum and testes

A punch or kick gives similar findings to a fall onto a hard object; this may be unintentional in rough play. The most likely injury is a contusion. The resultant swelling may make it difficult to decide whether this is a simple contusion or whether the testis has been damaged. Torsion of the testis, a ruptured corpus callosum, a hydrocoele or rupture of the testis can all occur. An ultrasound examination may help. Discussion with a surgeon is advised for scrotal and testicular injuries. Penetrating injuries can occur, for example, while climbing over a gate or railing. These must all be referred to a surgeon.

ANAL INJURIES

Minor injury to the anus due to an accident in childhood is very uncommon. All patients with anal and peri-anal injuries should therefore be referred for senior advice.

ASSOCIATED PATHOLOGY

Sometimes minor trauma can cause more severe effects if the area was already inflamed. This will potentially confuse your examination. These conditions commonly occur under the age of 6 years. Examples of such conditions include vulvovaginitis, psoriasis, streptococcal infection, candidiasis, threadworms, lichen sclerosus et atrophicus or inflammatory bowel disease.

CHAPTER 14

NON-ACCIDENTAL INJURY

INTRODUCTION

Sadly, any clinician treating minor injuries in children has to be aware of the possibility of non-accidental injury (NAI). You could be forgiven for thinking that paediatricians are perhaps obsessed by it, but delay in diagnosis is common, and making a diagnosis can be difficult. The repercussions of either a 'false negative' or 'false positive' diagnosis can be very damaging.

As well as minor injury, abused children may suffer major injury, sexual abuse or neglect. The profile of highly publicised cases can be misleading: news items focus on sequential 'missed opportunities' by professionals to detect repeated abuse, but this does not represent the broad spectrum of safeguarding issues we face in practice. An excellent evidence-based resource which has reviewed the world literature and captures the likelihood of an injury being abusive has been collated in recent years by the CORE INFO group.

 http://www.core-info.cardiff.ac.uk/reviews

Major inflicted injury occurs mainly in children under 1 year of age. Minor injuries may be inflicted, usually in older infants and preschool children, or may arise from lack of supervision (neglect). Among fractures from accidents, 85% occur in children over 5 years old, and 80% of abusive fractures occur in infants under 18 months old.

Both abusive injury and neglect are associated with risk factors in the family, such as social fragmentation, drug or alcohol misuse, or mental health problems in the adults closely associated with the child.

Virtually all urgent and emergency care facilities have a safeguarding/child protection policy. In the UK, there is a NICE (National Institute for Clinical Excellence) guideline called 'When to suspect child maltreatment', published in 2009.

https://www.nice.org.uk/guidance/cg89

Follow your local child protection policy at all times!

POINTERS TO NON-ACCIDENTAL INJURY

Frontline professionals need to have 'radar' for signs of NAI, and know what to do next. There may be clues in the history, the examination or the X-ray images, and sometimes it is just 'gut instinct' which prompts a deeper search for the truth.

At any time in your consultation there may be a pointer to NAI!

Senior and experienced medical and nursing colleagues usually have good 'radar', and will help make the decision whether to seek further information (finding out if there have been previous concerns about the family) or to seek an expert opinion (from a consultant paediatrician or social worker).

Neglect and poor supervision are much more common causes of welfare concerns than inflicted injury, and good judgement of the situation requires experience of both normal patterns of injury and of normal parenting. If you are not sure, ask your colleagues for their opinion.

Tips for history and examination
Consider NAI in the following circumstances:

- Story of the 'accident' is vague and lacks detail
- The story is variable and changes with each telling, e.g. at triage, with the doctor, in radiology

- There was a delay in seeking medical help
- History is not compatible with the injury observed
- History is not compatible with the child's developmental stage (e.g. rolled off a bed, aged 3 months)
- The patient is a non-mobile infant
- Unusual number of previous attendances with injuries or minor medical conditions
- History of violence or neglect amongst the rest of the family
- Child discloses abuse (this is unusual)
- Appearance of the child and/or interaction with the carers appears abnormal

In an infant who is not fully mobile and has an injury, you must consider NAI as part of your initial differential diagnosis!

When you listen to the history, it should flow naturally and with detail of the events, people's reactions and what happened next, unless there is a language barrier or the adults who have brought the child were not there at the time of the accident. Most of us could ask our parents to recall an accident from our childhood and still receive a detailed, blow-by-blow account, many years later. A friendly approach and open questioning is important in order to encourage this level of detail. The less information that you are given, the more suspicious you should be.

Be highly suspicious of injury with no explanation!

Have a low threshold for X-ray in children under 4 years. Children of this age group rarely sustain painful soft tissue injuries. If a limb persists in being painful, it may be fractured.

Building and balancing information

In many cases of inflicted injury or of neglect, you will reach a balanced opinion by putting together a 'jigsaw' of information and by talking with experienced colleagues. As well as information about the current injury (which may require you to speak to witnesses by telephone), you should seek a background risk profile of the family. Check if there is anything unusual in the child's address, next of kin and previous hospital attendances. Ask the family if they have a social worker involved with them. This is a useful question to ask during the initial assessment/triage phase.

Depending on your level of concern, you may want to telephone social care services to independently verify this. Consider speaking to the general practitioner (family doctor), who is ideally placed to flag any risk factors within the whole family. In the UK, preschool aged children have a named health visitor, who can usually provide information about parenting skills and the social situation. The majority of cases of abuse or neglect are diagnosed in this way, rather than being clear-cut from the outset.

Specific injuries suggestive of abuse

Certain injuries are highly suspicious of NAI. These include:

- A subdural haemorrhage or skull fracture without a high-impact head injury (e.g. fall from above head height; see Chapter 4)
- A spiral fracture of the humerus (see Chapter 7)
- Corner metaphyseal fractures of long-bones
- Fractures of different ages (the older fracture or callous formation may be picked up as an incidental finding alongside the new fracture)

Other injuries may happen either as a result of NAI or of accidents, for example:

- Fractured femur (usually an awkward landing or a twist)
- Spiral fracture of the tibia (a twisting mechanism should be described)
- Scalds and burns

A systematic review of injuries presenting to urgent and emergency care services found associations with NAI in the injuries listed in Table14.1.

Corner metaphyseal fractures are difficult to spot. They are highly suggestive of abuse and are thought to result from twisting the limb or shaking the child. They occur in children under the age of 4, typically those under 1 year. They are most common in the tibia.

Table 14.1 Fracture associations in children under 18 months with NAI (CORE INFO, http://www.core-info.cardiff.ac.uk/reviews).

- Multiple fractures are more common after physical abuse than after non-abusive traumatic injury.
- A child with multiple rib fractures has a 7 in 10 chance of having been abused.
- Multiple rib fractures are more common in abuse than in non-abuse.
- A child with a femoral fracture has a 1 in 3–4 chance of having been abused.
- Femoral fractures resulting from abuse are more commonly seen in children who are not yet walking.
- A child aged under 3 with a humeral fracture has a 1 in 2 chance of having been abused.
- Mid-shaft fractures of the humerus are more common in abuse than in non-abuse, whereas supracondylar fractures are more likely to have non-abusive causes.
- An infant or toddler with a skull fracture has a 1 in 3 chance of having been abused.
- Parietal and linear skull fractures are the most common type of skull fracture seen in abuse and non-abuse.
- No clear difference exists in the distribution of complex skull fractures between the two groups.

They occur due to shearing of the immature bone, which forms a ring of weakness under the rim of the metaphysis. This means they can be seen as a bucket handle or a corner depending on how the bone is viewed. The fracture's appearance can be transient as they can heal quickly without trace. Alternatively, they can heal with a periosteal reaction extending along the diaphysis of the bone. Figure 14.1 shows some examples, including the 'bucket-handle appearance'. Spiral fractures of the shaft of the humerus (Figure 14.2), and fractures of the shaft of the femur in children who have not yet started walking, are both fractures which are highly suggestive of abuse.

A subdural haemorrhage (Figure 14.3) can be caused either accidentally or from abuse. You will need to put the findings in context with the history (as discussed previously) and any risk factors for abuse. However, if injuries of two different ages are found, abuse is very likely.

Sometimes fractures can occur with minimal trauma, but this will be in the context of pathological fractures (abnormal bones). There are some

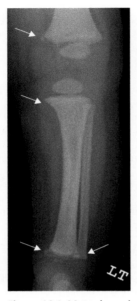

Figure 14.1 Metaphyseal corner and bucket-handle fractures.

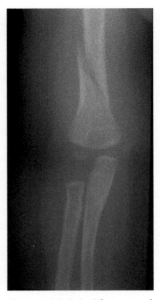

Figure 14.2 Spiral fracture of the shaft of the humerus in a 1-month-old baby due to non-accidental injury.

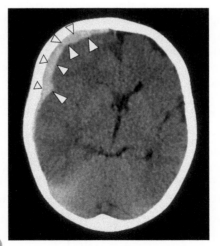

Figure 14.3 Acute subdural haemorrhage due to NAI.

Note the crescent-shaped fresh white haemorrhage on the right causing compression of the lateral ventricle and midline shift. Intracranial haematomas gradually become isodense to brain tissue over 2 weeks and eventually become the same density as cerebro-spinal fluid (CSF).

fragile bone diseases, such as osteogenesis imperfecta, and some children have osteoporosis – for example those who are wheelchair-bound. In this context, fractures suggestive of abuse may occur but actually not be secondary to abuse. This is one of the reasons why this is a specialist field and you should seek senior help, in order not to over- or under-diagnose abuse.

WHAT DO I DO IF I HAVE SOME CONCERN?

Do not be afraid to voice concern – you have a duty to do so. Spend time gathering information (as discussed earlier in the chapter), sharing your concern with colleagues and following your organisation's child protection policy. In many situations, it is best to admit the child to the hospital under the care of a paediatrician, to allow time to gather more information, get second opinions from experienced colleagues and keep the child safe from further harm. You can keep things calm by not stating an opinion, and simply saying that you are asking for a specialist opinion, as your role is only to make an initial assessment of the injury. Playing down your role in this way is something the parents cannot reasonably be upset about.

Further assessment of the child will then take place in a safe environment. This will likely include (for children under 2 years) a 'skeletal survey', which is a detailed X-ray series of many parts of the body in order to detect occult fractures, which are common in NAI. Head CT and spinal MRI imaging may also be done at this stage, looking for occult trauma.

GOOD RECORD-KEEPING

Your records should reflect the level of detail of questions that you have actually asked, especially in the younger (more at-risk) children. For example:

- A precise mechanism of injury. When? How? Why? Landing onto what surface? Landing in what position?
- The circumstances. Who was there? How much pain was the child in? How and when was medical help sought?

Be clear in your record of your examination:

- Document shapes and sizes of the injury and use diagrams when possible
- In non-mobile children or any child where you have a possible suspicion of NAI, examine the whole child, fully unclothed

Be specific about all conversations with other professionals:

- Date and time of each conversation, name and contact number of the other party and a record of your agreed outcome

Ensure the child's notes have all relevant demographic information. This matters if things escalate in the future, or for example, if the parents abscond with the child before medical treatment is finished. Details of siblings will help the general practitioner or social worker trace all relevant family information.

PRACTICAL PROCEDURES

INTRODUCTION

There is a wide range of practical procedures needed for the management of minor injuries – many are not well described or taught in conventional medical or nursing education. Because young children are less likely to cooperate with therapeutic procedures such as suturing or foreign body removal, these are more likely to be performed under general anaesthesia than in adult practice. This is less likely if the team has good communication skills (see Chapter 2) and good practical skills.

EXAMINATION OF EARS, NOSE AND THROAT

Many children dislike examination of their ears, nose and throat (ENT). The following clinches are designed to prevent the strongest of children escaping! This is important to both prevent the child being hurt by being poked by your equipment, and to make the examination as rapid as possible. If a parent loses their grip, it may be better to employ the skills of an experienced nurse.

Before you start, show the child your auriscope light. This ensures they feel they are not being 'pounced upon' and the light can help engage them.

Ears

Sit the child sideways on the adult's lap, asking them to 'cuddle' the child with one of their hands holding the child's arm, and their other hand over the child's head, as shown in Figure 15.1. The child is turned the opposite way for examination of the other side.

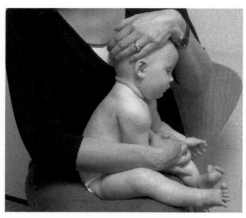

 Figure 15.1 **Ear examination.**

Nose and throat

Make sure you are in good light or use the light of the auriscope or a pen torch. Sit the child on the adult's lap, facing you. The adult is asked to put one of their arms across both of the child's, and the other hand across the child's forehead, as shown in Figure 15.2, with the head tilted slightly backwards. In order to get a view of the throat, try to get the tongue depressor between the teeth. If the jaw shuts, persistent, firm pressure will result in the child eventually giving way. You can then advance the tongue depressor onto the tongue.

SLINGS

Broad arm sling

Using a triangular bandage, place it across the chest as shown in Figure 15.3. Take the bottom corner up to the shoulder on the affected side, and tie a knot at the side of the neck with the remaining corner (Figure 15.4). At the elbow, bring the free flap across and pin to the front of the sling (Figure 15.5).

 Video 15.1 Application of broad arm sling: https://youtu.be/s977N22Cbs8

High arm sling

Using a triangular bandage, place it across the chest, over the injured arm, as shown in Figure 15.6. Take the bottom corner under the arm, up

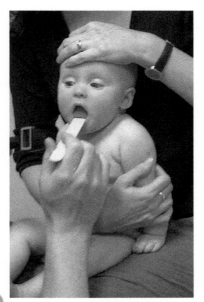

Figure 15.2 Throat examination.

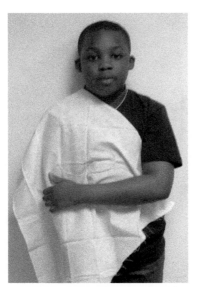

Figure 15.3 Application of a broad arm sling: Step 1.

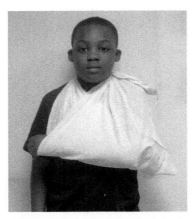

 Figure 15.4 **Application of a broad arm sling: Step 2.**

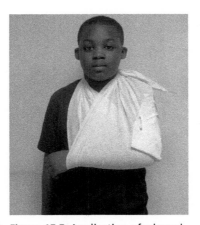

 Figure 15.5 **Application of a broad arm sling: Step 3.**

to the shoulder on the affected side and tie a knot to the side of the neck (Figure 15.7). Tie and secure as for broad arm sling.

 Video 15.2 Application of high arm sling: https://youtu.be/FJiaLZd2jrM

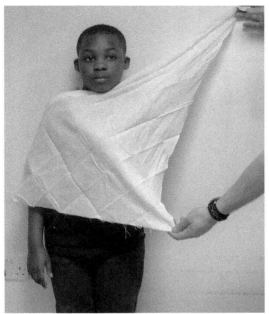

Figure 15.6 Application of a high arm sling: Step 1.

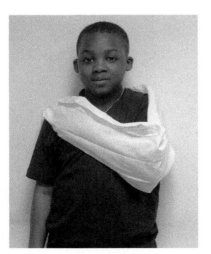

Figure 15.7 Application of a high arm sling: Step 2.

'Collar and cuff'

Place a foam sling ('collar and cuff') or a long bandage around the neck, keeping one side long and the hand partially elevated. Wrap the short end around the wrist on the affected side. Bring the long end across, meeting above the wrist, and tie around all three layers (Figure 15.8). Then cut off any excess foam or bandage.

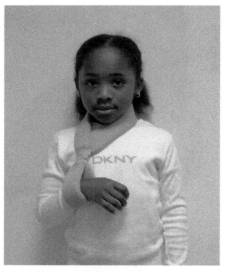

 Figure 15.8 **Application of a collar and cuff.**

 Video 15.3 Application of collar and cuff: https://youtu.be/qULS5K50OBQ.

NEIGHBOUR STRAPPING

Place some folded gauze between the affected finger and a neighbouring finger, to prevent the skin rubbing. Then place tapes across the proximal and middle phalanges, avoiding the PIPJ and DIPJ, to permit movement of the joints, as shown in Figure 15.9.

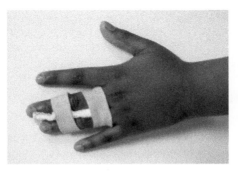

 Figure 15.9 Application of neighbour strapping.

 Video 15.4 Application of neighbor strapping: https://youtu.be/VGKJa2RP0QQ

An alternative to neighbour strapping is the Bedford Splint.

 Video 15.5 Application of Bedford splint: https://youtu.be/I3hKEVRs358.

To immobilise just one finger, a Zimmer splint is an alternative treatment.

 Video 15.6 Application of Zimmer splint: https://youtu.be/JKtA9JaYrnU.

BLANKET WRAP' FOR IMMOBILISATION

It is sometimes easier to wrap the child up to get a very short procedure on the head or face done quickly, by stopping arm and leg movement. Most parents understand that for a quick procedure, it is better to achieve what you want to do safely, and in the shortest time possible. However, if a child is really struggling and upset, you need to change tactics, in order to avoid psychological harm.

 If the procedure is going to take longer than a minute or so, consider procedural sedation (see Chapter 2)!

First lay the child on a blanket. Then wrap one side of the blanket diagonally across the child, incorporating the body and one arm, as shown in, then wrap the other side around to include the other arm, leaving only the head out (Figure 15.10).

FOREIGN BODIES

Removal of nasal foreign body

'The kissing technique' is a humane little technique for a nasal foreign body which unfortunately is not well known, and in the majority of cases avoids progression to instrumentation or general anaesthesia. The parent tells the child that mummy/daddy is going to give him/her 'a big kiss'.
Step 1: Ask the parent to sit the child on their lap sideways on, cuddled up to their chest. Have tissue ready to catch the expelled foreign body!
Step 2: The parent occludes the unaffected nostril with a finger. Step 3: They seal their mouth over the child's and deliver a short, sharp puff of breath. If a parent is unable to understand this, a bag-valve mask device over the mouth can be used instead.

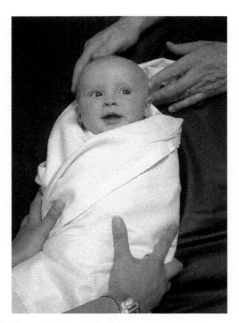

 Figure 15.10 A blanket wrap for short procedures.

Video 15.7 'Kissing technique' for a nasal foreign body: https://youtu.be/
YM73eaLnmWk

The force of the air going up through the nasopharynx forces the foreign
body down the nostril. Sometimes more than one puff is necessary. The
child usually doesn't mind, if you make a game out of it. If this technique
fails, then a blanket wrap may be necessary to remove the foreign body
with some fine forceps. If it is difficult to retrieve, refer to ENT because
you may hurt the child, and risk further damage or aspiration.

Removal of a foreign body in the ear

There are many techniques for removing a foreign body in the ear. Small
right-angled forceps (Tilley's forceps or crocodile forceps) may be used for
pieces of paper or cotton wool. Alternatively, suction may be applied by
using a fine suction catheter. Also, irrigation using warm water or olive oil
may be used for small objects (e.g. insects). For seeds and beans do not use
irrigation, as the foreign body may swell.

A Jobson Horne probe (straight with a loop at the end) is needed for
rounded objects such as beads; if you do not have one of these you can
straighten out a paper clip, leaving a bend in the middle. Make an angled
'hoop' at one end by bending it back on itself, taking care to ensure the
sharp end does not protrude, as shown in Figure 15.11. This shape is ideal
for manoeuvring behind the object, then scooping it out. For embedded
earrings, see the section 'Auricular nerve block'.

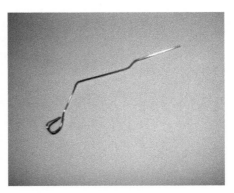

 Figure 15.11 A paper clip bent into a scoop
to retrieve rounded objects.

Removal of a foreign body in the eye

These may be seen in a good light on the surface of the cornea with the naked eye, or may require a slit lamp to magnify the cornea. Alternatively, the foreign body can be stuck under the upper or lower eyelid, or may have gone, leaving an allergic reaction or an abrasion.

Anaesthetic drops are usually needed. These sting, so the child will need a lot of reassurance; younger children will often need to be referred to an ophthalmologist. Once the drops are in, get the child to look in all directions. If you cannot see anything, hold the eyelids wide. If you still see nothing, get the child to look at the floor and using a cotton wool bud, evert the upper eyelid.

To remove the foreign body a cotton bud soaked in water can be dragged across the tissues to lift it off. If this does not work, in a cooperative child the 'scoop' of the bevel of a standard IV needle can be used to dislodge it, keeping the needle sideways to the eye, ideally under the magnification of a slit lamp. This is best not attempted until you have been taught the technique.

Video 15.8 Removal of a corneal foreign body: https://youtu.be/uw2VTvsQcYw

Irrigation of eyes

Unlike commercially available 'eye baths', copious water is actually required to relieve symptoms from chemicals or dust. This requires a litre or more of normal saline IV solution, run through an IV giving set or using specialist irrigation equipment, and run as a steady stream over the eye(s), with the child lying on their back with their head over the side of the couch or ideally, backwards over a sink. Topical anaesthetic drops are needed before you start, to help keep the eye open. These sting, so the child will need a little cajoling.

REDUCTION OF A 'PULLED ELBOW'

This common injury is sustained when a toddler is pulled by the hand (see Chapter 7). You must explain what you are about to do to the parent, in the most reassuring terms, and warn them that the child will cry.

Make sure the mechanism of injury is classical, and the child is the right age group, before attempting reduction without prior X-ray!

Step 1: Sit the child on the parent's lap, sideways on. Step 2: Put one thumb over the head of the radius and with your other hand, hold the child's hand. Step 3: Fully supinate and pronate the forearm in the bent position. You may feel a click, either beneath your thumb, or transmitted down to the hand. Step 4: If not, move quickly to doing the same (supination, pronation) with the arm in full extension, then return the arm to its original position – the click may be felt at either stage. Step 5: Whether or not a click was felt, leave room at this stage to allow the child to settle down and play with some toys, to see if they start using the arm. Review the child after 10 minutes. See Chapter 7 for further management.

Video 15.9 Reduction of a pulled elbow: https://youtu.be/x8I7St8_2Kw

TREPHINING A NAIL

Crush injuries to fingertips are common, and may cause a subungual haematoma (see Chapter 8). Trephining the nail releases the blood and is a satisfying procedure because of the instant relief of symptoms. To do this, the nail is literally melted by a hot metal wire, to make a hole through which the blood drains (beware, it often spurts out like a fountain!). If performed quickly and efficiently, there is only a second or so of pain at most; get a second member of staff to hold the child's hand down to prevent sudden withdrawal.

Your place of work should ideally have a purpose-made battery-operated device in which a fine wire heats up, but if not, a paper clip can be used. A needle will do the job, but is at increased risk of penetrating the nailbed and causing further pain or harm. When the metal is red hot, puncture the nail with one firm, swift action, withdrawing quickly. Do not be put off by burning and hissing!

The paper clip technique involves straightening out one side of a paper clip and applying some elastoplast to the remaining clip to prevent you burning your fingers as it heats up. Heat the straight part in a flame (e.g. a paraffin oil lamp or cigarette lighter), then proceed as above.

Video 15.10 Trephining of a nail: https://youtu.be/diO67RG3w0k

WOUND MANAGEMENT

Wound irrigation

See Chapter 3 for advice about wound management. To clean a wound adequately, irrigation with copious quantities of water is the most important principle, to decrease the bacterial load. For example, if you dilute a tenth of a tenth of a tenth (i.e. 10 ml three times over), the bacteria are diluted by 1,000.

Infiltrate the wound with local anaesthetic if necessary. Place the affected part on a good thickness of absorbent towels. Use a 20 ml or 50 ml syringe and a large bowl of water or saline to repeatedly flush inside the wound, or use a litre of IV saline, directing the flow through a standard IV giving set.

Video 15.11 Wound irrigation: https://youtu.be/5VE8-DXG-hc

Adhesive strips and glue

Adhesive strips such as Steri-Strips and tissue glue provide equal, if not better, cosmetic outcomes than sutures for many wounds. It all depends on the tension across the wound, which is only partly related to its depth, but significantly related to wound length and the direction of the wound to Langer's lines (see Chapter 3).

Both adhesive strips and glue are probably of similar efficacy and both may be used together if a wound needs good support. Adhesive strips cannot be used on hairy areas; tissue glue cannot be used near the eyes.

Applying adhesive strips

These should be laid perpendicular to the wound, bringing a small amount of tension to the wound edges to ensure adequate opposition but not bunching up the edges. For children, it is worth laying extra strips at 90°, over either end of the main strips. Tincture of benzoin can help stick them down, especially if the skin is sweaty or the wound moist, but make sure this does not go into the wound. Circumferential strips should not be applied around fingertips; apply them longitudinally to allow for swelling. Steri-Strips should remain in place for a day or so longer than sutures – i.e. 5 days if not under tension and a week if on a mobile part of the body.

Video 15.12 Application of adhesive strips: https://youtu.be/6oXWYtqc-VQ

Applying tissue glue

Tissue glue is not totally painless – there is burning during the exothermic reaction as it hardens. However, as a concept it seems to appeal to children, thus overcoming their apprehension. N.B. Sterile gloves stick easily to glue!

Take care only to place the glue as a seal over the top of the wound. If it drips between the wound edges, it will have the opposite effect of preventing healing. The glue will dissolve after several washes so advise the family to keep the wound dry for 5 days then treat as normal, and it will disappear over the next 2 weeks.

 Care must be taken to avoid the eyes!

If any glue is dropped near the eyes stop and wipe immediately with a wet swab. If this does not work, it will gradually come off over the coming days, but further attempts at removal before this time are likely to result in more damage. If any glue enters the eye, refer immediately to ophthalmology.

 Video 15.13 Application of wound adhesive: https://youtu.be/vc-CGAbzDK4

Local infiltration of anaesthesia

If there is no regional block for a particular area (see 'Regional anaesthesia (nerve blocks)'), anaesthetic agents may be infiltrated locally. The choice of anaesthetic is explained in Table 15.1. Infiltration of local anaesthesia is generally very safe, but overdose may result in facial tingling, cardiac arrhythmias and seizures.

 If the toxic dose of local anaesthetic is likely to be exceeded, the child will need general anaesthesia for wound repair!

 Will the child cooperate or will they need sedation or general anaesthesia (see Chapter 2)?

Table 15.1 **Choice of local anaesthetic agents**

Drug	Toxic dose	Indications
1% Lignocaine	3 mg/kg (= 0.3 mL/kg)	Local wound infiltration. Onset 2–3 min. Offset variable but usually < 1 hour
2% Lignocaine	3 mg/kg (= 0.15 mL/kg)	Small volume so useful for finger and auricular blocks.
Lignocaine 1% with Adrenaline (1:200,000)	6 mg/kg of lignocaine component (=0.6 mL/kg)	Vascular areas e.g. face, scalp. Avoid in end-organs, e.g. fingers, penis, pinna.
Bupivacaine	2 mg/kg (0.4 mL/kg of 0.5% solution)	Longer acting than lignocaine. Onset 5 mins. Offset 1–4 hours. Often used for regional blocks.

After cleaning, inject anaesthetic into the wound edges using a blue (23 gauge) or orange (25 gauge) needle, passing the needle straight into the subcutaneous tissues through the wound edge rather than through the intact skin, which is more painful. Slow injection will decrease stinging. A dental needle is best, if available. Inject further anaesthetic through the area you have just anaesthetised, waiting half a minute if there are few injections and the child is cooperative.

Video 15.14 Injecting local anaesthetic: https://youtu.be/7mRJqM29CRA

Suturing

For a full description of the indications for, and pitfalls regarding, suturing, see Chapter 3. When choosing suture material, consider using absorbable sutures, which is a useful option for avoiding suture removal in children. Find out what your local policy is, since the evidence base for equivalence to absorbable sutures is weak. The size of suture depends on the amount of tension or wear and tear over the area, but should be the smallest size possible, e.g. 3-0 or 4-0 for scalps, 4-0 or 5-0 for limbs and 5-0 or 6-0 for faces.

Think twice before suturing a wound on the face – are you sufficiently skilled?

This is the technique for inserting interrupted sutures, the commonest approach for wound closure for traumatic wounds. Step 1: Pick up the needle with the suture holder, as shown in Figure 15.12. The needle holder should be placed about two thirds of the way back along the needle. Step 2: Introduce the needle to the skin at 90° and aim vertically down to include sufficient tissue to provide support for the suture, and avoid tension on the wound, as shown in Figure 15.13. Hold the tissue with forceps, avoiding crushing the edge of the wound. Push the needle through, following the curve of the needle. Pull most of the thread through, allowing a small length to remain for tying. Pick this end up with your needle holder in your other hand.

Step 3: Tie a triple knot to secure the suture. Now pick up the long needle end of the thread and wrap it twice around the needle holder clockwise, as shown in Figure 15.14. Without letting go, let the thread slide off the needle holder and pull it tight to form a knot, as shown in Figure 15.15. Do not leave the knot over the middle of the wound, but bring it to the side. Ensure that the wound edges are not inverted, everted or under tension. This leads to scarring. Step 4: Repeat, wrapping anti-clockwise once around the needle holder and tie. Step 5: The same but wrap clockwise again. Cut the ends long enough to be identified easily and permit grasping when removing.

 Video 15.15 Suturing: https://youtu.be/QeBxTubhHOo

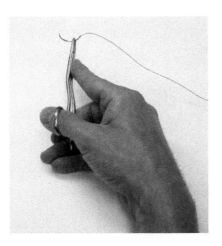

 Figure 15.12 The correct position for holding a needle.

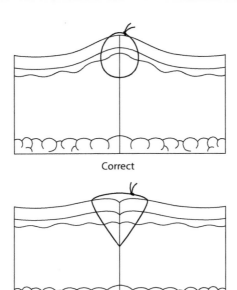

Correct

Incorrect

 Figure 15.13 A cross-section of skin tissues demonstrating correct placement of a suture.

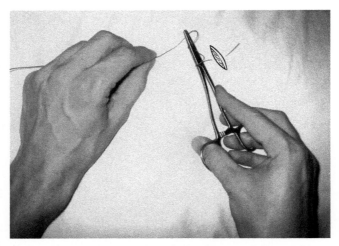

Figure 15.14 Wrapping the suture thread around the needle holder.

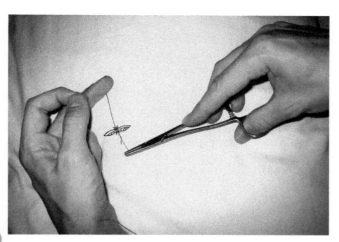

 Figure 15.15 **Tying a knot.**

Applying dressings

Keeping dressings on children is a challenge! The actual wound dressing you use can be whatever your local practice is, but keeping it in place for a few days, not to undo all your good work, is challenging. A 'belt and braces' approach for toddlers and some older children is worthwhile. For the most part use common sense, such as using the most adhesive dressings or tape that you have. There are certain areas of the body where little techniques handed down through generations of nurses are useful to know, such as the hand. These are difficult to describe in text but the online version of this book contains some videos to help you.

 Video 15.16 Application of hand dressing in small child: https://youtu.be/jHGaBtWlhN8

REGIONAL ANAESTHESIA (NERVE BLOCKS)

Techniques of regional anaesthesia are usually easy to learn and once mastered, can be very satisfying. Injection of anaesthetic away from the affected site is well tolerated by children, and the side effects of intravenous analgesia are avoided.

tal block

The four digital nerves are distributed around the phalanx as shown in Figure 15.16. Inject 1 ml of 2% lignocaine as close to the bone as possible, along two perpendicular sides, aspirating before injecting. Repeat on the other side.

Metacarpal block

An alternative to the digital block is a metacarpal block. This carries the advantage of a single injection, rather than two, and possibly better anaesthesia of the dorsum of the finger. 3 ml of 1% lignocaine is injected where the metacarpal neck becomes the head, in the palm. The dotted lines on Figure 15.17 show where to inject.

Auricular nerve block

This block is invaluable for procedures on the lower half of the pinna, in particular for removing embedded earrings. The earlobe is often swollen and may be infected and extremely tender; injecting anaesthetic into the earlobe is very painful and difficult. However, injecting away from the ear is usually well tolerated. The block works up to around halfway up the pinna. It blocks branches of the greater auricular and auriculotemporal nerves.

Using about 4 ml of 2% lignocaine, the needle enters the skin 1 cm below where the earlobe joins the face (near the angle of the jaw, as shown in Figure 15.18). Direct half the volume anteriorly towards the tragus, and half posteriorly, back towards the mastoid.

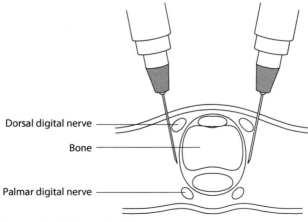

Dorsal digital nerve

Bone

Palmar digital nerve

Figure 15.16 **The digital block technique.**

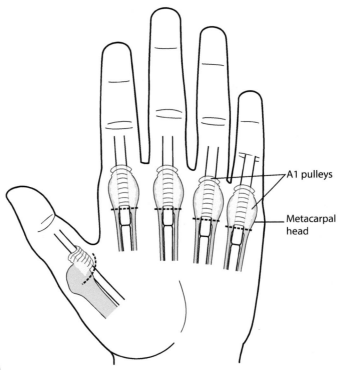

Figure 15.17 Technique for a metacarpal block.

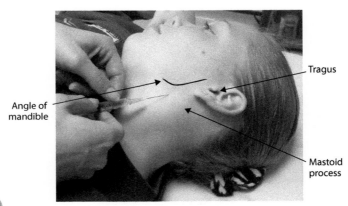

Figure 15.18 The inferior auricular block technique.

A-ARTICULAR BLOCK FOR SHOULDER DISLOCATION

This is a very useful block which reduces pain in a dislocated shoulder. With this block, you may be able to reduce the dislocation with either no additional analgesia, if you go slowly (see Chapter 7), or with Entonox only. It is good to avoid procedural sedation, if you can.

Insert 15-20 mL of 1% lidocaine (15 mL in a child smaller than an adult or 20 mL for full adult size) via a 20 mL syringe with a 21g needle. Insert the needle below the acromion, aiming 90 degrees to the skin so that it enters the large space created by the dislocation.

Withdraw to check for blood. If you see blood this is most likely due to a capsule tear than because you have entered a vessel. Reposition your needle and if the same happens, you can be sure that it is capsular blood, so you can continue and inject.

Inject the full volume over 20 seconds. The block takes 10-15 minutes to work.

See Figure 15.19 for landmarks.

Femoral nerve block and 'three in one' nerve block

These blocks are used to provide analgesia for a fractured shaft of femur. The block should be performed before X-ray or application of traction. A femoral nerve block uses a syringe and needle directed vertically downwards. A 'three in one' block, via an intravenous cannula instead of a needle, uses the same initial anatomical landmarks, but is placed higher, before the trifurcation of the femoral, obturator and lateral cutaneous nerve of the thigh; it is a less painful technique, and avoids inadvertently hitting the nerve with a needle.

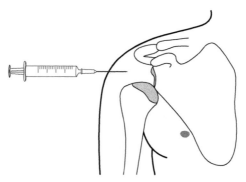

Figure 15.19 Intra-articular anaesthetic injection of the shoulder for dislocation.

These blocks take about 20 minutes to work, so IV morphine or intranasal opiate may be required in the interim!

Femoral nerve block

Use 0.5% bupivacaine with a volume of around 2 mg/kg (i.e. 0.4 ml/kg). Draw up the anaesthetic in a syringe, then attach a 21 Ch needle. Partially abduct the leg and locate the femoral pulse and the inguinal ligament. For a child under 8 years old, enter the skin 1 cm lateral to the pulse, just below the inguinal ligament, and for children over 8 years, enter 2 cm lateral to the pulse. Aim directly downwards as far as you would for arterial or venous sampling, aspirating regularly. If there is no flushback, slowly inject the anaesthetic.

Modified femoral nerve block ('three in one' block)

Use the same volume of anaesthetic and landmarks as for the femoral block, but use a 20 Ch cannula. Direct the cannula in line with the leg, at 45° to the skin, as shown in Figure 15.20. Once it is halfway in, try to advance the cannula over the needle. If you are in the right place (a potential space overlying the psoas fascia) it should advance freely. Check there is no flushback, then attach your syringe and inject the anaesthetic. This should inject freely, as if into a vein.

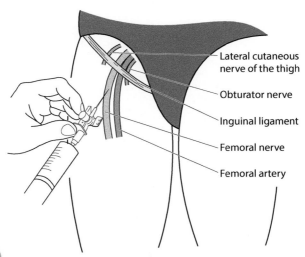

Figure 15.20 The 'three in one' block technique.

blocks

The nerve distribution to the foot is individually quite variable, but installation of a block is much easier than local infiltration into the sole of the foot.

These blocks take 10 to 15 minutes to work.

Dorsum of the foot
Infiltrate 1 ml 2% lignocaine either side of the dorsalis pedis artery, as shown in Figure 15.21. This anaesthetises the medial plantar nerve. Aim to puncture the skin only once, with repositioning of the needle by withdrawing slightly.

Medial border of the sole
Infiltrate 1 ml 2% lignocaine either side of the posterior tibial artery, behind the medial malleolus, as shown in Figure 15.22, using the same technique as above. This anaesthetises the posterior tibial nerve.

Lateral border of the sole
Infiltrate 3–5 ml of 1% lignocaine between the lateral malleolus and the Achilles tendon, in a line, a few centimetres higher than the tip of the lateral malleolus (Figure 15.23). This anaesthetises the sural nerve.

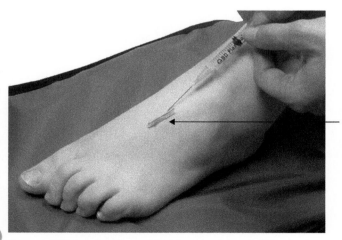

Figure 15.21 Landmarks for blocking the dorsum of the foot.

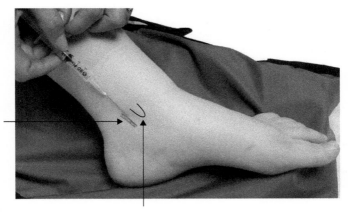

Figure 15.22 Landmarks for blocking the medial border of the sole.

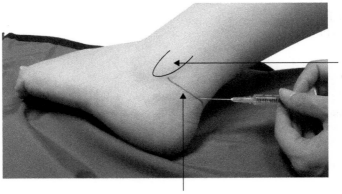

Figure 15.23 Landmarks for blocking the lateral border of the sole.

INDEX

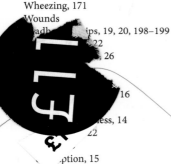